Management of the Difficult Airway

A Handbook for Surgeons

Management of the Difficult Airway

A Handbook for Surgeons

Edited by

Jerome W Thompson, MD, MBA
Professor and Chairman
Department of Otolaryngology – Head and Neck Surgery
University of Tennessee Health Science Center
LeBonheur Children's Medical Center
St Jude Children's Research Hospital
Memphis, Tennessee
USA

Francisco Vieira, MD
Professor of Otolaryngology – Head and Neck Surgery
Department of Otolaryngology – Head and Neck Surgery
University of Tennessee
Memphis, Tennessee
USA

Michael J Rutter, MBChB, FRACS
Professor of Pediatric Otolaryngology – Head and Neck Surgery
Division of Pediatric Otolaryngology – Head and Neck Surgery
Cincinnati Children's Hospital Medical Center
Department of Otolaryngology – Head and Neck Surgery
University of Cincinnati College of Medicine
Cincinnati, Ohio
USA

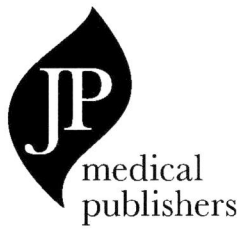

JP
medical
publishers

London • Philadelphia • Panama City • New Delhi

Published by JP Medical Ltd, 83 Victoria Street, London, SW1H 0HW, UK
Tel: +44 (0)20 3170 8910   Fax: +44 (0)20 3008 6180
Email: info@jpmedpub.com   Web: www.jpmedpub.com

ISBN: 978-1-909836-05-1

British Library Cataloguing in Publication Data
A catalogue record for this book is available from the British Library

Library of Congress Cataloging in Publication Data
A catalog record for this book is available from the Library of Congress

Publisher:	Richard Furn
Associate Publisher	Geoff Greenwood
Development Editor:	Gavin Smith
Editorial Assistant	Katie Pattullo
Design:	Designers Collective Ltd

Preface

Surgeons and critical care physicians are frequently faced with a serious airway emergency as part of their daily practice. Too often however, many years have elapsed since their residency or there are gaps in their knowledge due to the varying quality of specialty training. No patient should die because of these shortcomings.

The purpose of *Management of the Difficult Airway: A Handbook for Surgeons* is to enable surgeons to rapidly review the latest best practice in airway management. The structure of the text is designed to provide an accessible reference for clinicians with different levels of training and skills and the requisite information to assist with life-saving efforts in a critical situation.

We have gathered leading experts to provide a concise but thorough resource for board review, recertification and for use during residency training. While focusing primarily on the needs of the surgical population, the book is also relevant to other emergency healthcare providers, for use in training and in preparation for proficiency exams.

After an introductory chapter that provides a brief history of the evolution of airway management, chapter 2 describes the anatomic structures of the airway, providing the clinician with a common nomenclature for use when discussing disease, injury and interventions. Chapter 3 shows the value that radiological imaging can bring to the conceptualization – so invaluable prior to interventions – of structures and pathology. Chapter 4 gives insights into the resources available to our anesthesia colleagues in the management of difficult airways. Chapter 5 discusses the indications for instrument intervention, since no action is sometimes better than an ill advised one. Chapter 6 explains the emergency surgical management of the airway in urgent situations, while chapter 7 provides a comprehensive update on the latest equipment available to clinicians. Chapters 8 and 9 give an in-depth discussion of pediatric airway management – challenging because of the different disease processes and techniques involved. Chapter 10 presents the EXIT procedure and the extreme but necessary life-saving technique for use in neonates. Chapter 11 discusses the reconstruction of the damaged or inadequately developed airway while chapter 12 presents the new technique of balloon dilation for narrowed airways. Chapter 13 describes the unique problems presented in the management of airways invaded or destroyed by cancer. Chapter 14 concludes the text with an overview of ICU management of the critical airway.

We hope *Management of the Difficult Airway: A Handbook for Surgeons* helps our readers and makes a difference to the care of their patients.

Jerome Thompson
Francisco Vieira
Michael J Rutter
August 2015

Contents

Contributors

Karthik Balakrishnan, MD, MPH
Senior Associate Consultant, Pediatric
Otolaryngology
Department of Otorhinolaryngology
Eugenio Litta Children's Center
Mayo Clinic
Rochester, Minnesota
USA

Howard R Bromley, MD, MBA, FACPM
Clinical Associate Professor of
Anesthesiology, Critical Care and Pain
Management
University of Tennessee Health Sciences
Center
Memphis, Tennessee
USA

Martin A Croce, MD, FACS
Professor of Surgery
Department of Surgery
University of Tennessee Health Science
Center
Memphis, Tennessee
USA

Karuna Dewan, MD
Clinical Instructor and Laryngology Fellow
UCLA School of Medicine
Department of Head and Neck Surgery
Los Angeles, California
USA

Adryan A Emion, CRNA, DNP
Lead CRNA
Department of Anesthesia
University of Tennessee Regional One
Physicians
Memphis, Tennessee
USA

Amado X Freire, MD, MPH
Professor and Division Chief, Pulmonary,
Critical Care and Sleep Medicine
Department of Medicine
University of Tennessee Health Science
Center
Memphis, Tennessee
USA

Jonathan P Giurintano, MD
House Officer
Department of Otolaryngology – Head and
Neck Surgery
University of Tennessee Health Science
Center
Memphis, Tennessee
USA

R Ian Gray, MD
Assistant Professor of Neuroradiology
Department of Radiology
University of Tennessee, College of
Medicine
Memphis, Tennessee
USA

Catherine K Hart, MD
Assistant Professor of Pediatric
Otolaryngology – Head and Neck Surgery
Division of Pediatric Otolaryngology –
Head and Neck Surgery
Cincinnati Children's Hospital Medical
Center
Department of Otolaryngology – Head and
Neck Surgery
University of Cincinnati College of
Medicine
Cincinnati, Ohio
USA

Jennifer D McLevy, MD
Assistant Professor of Pediatric
Otolaryngology
Department of Otolaryngology
University of Tennessee
Memphis, Tennessee
USA

Luis C Murillo, MD, D-AASM, FCCP
Associate Professor
Adult Cystic Fibrosis Program Director
Pulmonary, Critical Care and Sleep
Medicine
University of Tennessee Health Science
Center
Memphis, Tennessee
USA

Kathleen G Ransom, MS, BS, RRT
Registered Respiratory Therapist
Department of Respiratory Therapy
Methodist North Hospital
Memphis, Tennessee
USA

Michael J Rutter, MBChB, FRACS
Professor of Pediatric Otolaryngology –
Head and Neck Surgery
Division of Pediatric Otolaryngology – Head
and Neck Surgery
Cincinnati Children's Hospital Medical
Center
Department of Otolaryngology – Head and
Neck Surgery
University of Cincinnati College of Medicine
Cincinnati, Ohio
USA

Sandeep Samant, MD
Professor, Department of Otolaryngology
Northwestern University
Department of Otolaryngology
Feinberg School of Medicine
Chicago, Illinois
USA

Sridhar Shankar, MD, MBA
Professor of Radiology
Department of Radiology
University of Tennessee
Memphis, Tennessee
USA

Kerry C Snyder, CRNA, DNP
Chief CRNA, Lead CRNA Trauma
Anesthesia
UT Regional One Physicians
Memphis, Tennessee
USA

Rose Mary Stocks, MD
Professor, Department of Otolaryngology
LeBonheur Children's Medical Center
St Jude Children's Research Hospital
Memphis, Tennessee
USA

Jerome W Thompson, MD, MBA
Professor and Chairman
Department of Otolaryngology – Head and
Neck Surgery
University of Tennessee Health Science
Center
LeBonheur Children's Medical Center
St Jude Children's Research Hospital
Memphis, Tennessee
USA

Jared J Tompkins, MD
Resident Physician
Department of Otolaryngology – Head and
Neck Surgery
The University of Tennessee Health Science
Center
Memphis, Tennessee
USA

R Mario Vera, MD
Assistant Professor of Surgery
Michael E. DeBakey Department of Surgery
Baylor College of Medicine
Houston, Texas
USA

Francisco Vieira, MD
Professor of Otolaryngology – Head and
Neck Surgery
Department of Otolaryngology – Head and
Neck Surgery
University of Tennessee
Memphis, Tennessee
USA

Joshua W Wood MD
Department of Otolaryngology – Head and
Neck Surgery
University of Tennessee Health Science
Center
Memphis, Tennessee
USA

Christina J Yang, MD
Assistant Professor of Pediatric
Otolaryngology – Head and Neck Surgery
Department of Otorhinolaryngology – Head
and Neck Surgery
Montefiore Medical Center and Albert
Einstein College of Medicine
Bronx, New York
USA

A brief history of airway management

Jerome W Thompson, Francisco Vieira

Early history

In recorded history, the tracheotomy is one of the oldest-known surgical procedures, first portrayed on Egyptian tablets in about 3600 BC (Jones 2009). In approximately 2000 BC, references can be found to tracheotomy in the *Rig Veda*, the ancient sacred Hindu text.

Tracheostomy is mentioned in the Egyptian Ebers Papyrus in 1550 BC. In the Greco-Roman Era, Hippocrates condemned tracheotomy, citing a threat to carotid arteries in 400 BC (Stock 1987). Galen, in about 131 AD, elucidated laryngeal and tracheal anatomy, localizing voice production to the larynx. He defined laryngeal innervation, and understood the importance of the trachea and lungs when he used a bellows to inflate lungs of dead animals. Asclepiades of Persia and Antyllus are both credited with early tracheotomies that would be familiar to modern physicians in 100 AD (Jones 2009). In 400 AD, the Susruta Samhita documents tracheotomy as an accepted therapy in India.

In 1308 AD, Dante declared that tracheotomy was 'a suitable punishment for a sinner in the depths of the Inferno.' Antonio Musa Brasavola, an Italian physician, performed the first well-documented successful tracheotomy in 1546 (**Figure 1.1**).

The 1700s

George Martine, who lived from 1702 to 1743, developed the inner cannula for tracheostomy tubes.

The 1800s

Arguably the most famous and significant use of the tracheotomy in the 1800s was upon Crown Prince Frederick of Germany, son-in-law of Queen Victoria, and brother of the younger future Kaiser Wilhelm. It is thought that his death was a possible contributor to World War I. Dr Morell Mackenzie popularized the laryngoscope to treat diseases of the larynx. The daughter of Queen Victoria requested that Dr Mackenzie travel from London to see her husband who had a laryngeal lesion and required a tracheostomy. The Crown Prince eventually died of laryngeal cancer, and, as foreigners, Mackenzie and the Princess were blamed. Prince Wilhelm became the Kaiser at a very young age and played a major role in the initiation of the World War I.

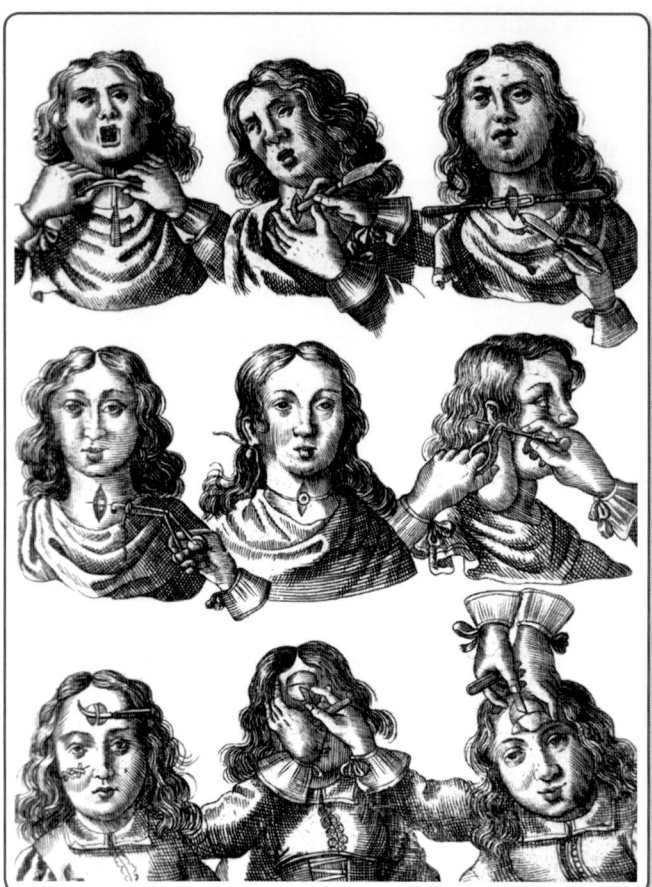

Figure 1.1 Engraving, Armamentarium chirurgicum bipartitum, 1660. The first five images shown in this engraving depict the tracheotomy procedure.

The 1900s

Chevalier Jackson is considered the father of modern laryngoscopy and bronchoscopy. His work reduced the risks involved in a tracheotomy and refined the techniques used in tracheotomies and their aftercare (Jackson 1909). He essentially invented the modern science of endoscopy of the upper airway and esophagus, using hollow tubes with small direct current electric light bulb illumination. He also developed methods for safely and effectively removing foreign bodies from the esophagus and the airway.

History of mask ventilation and intubation

Obstruction of the airway was a poorly understood phenomenon prior to 1874. Airway management amounted to opening the mouth with a wooden screw and drawing the tongue forward with a forceps or a steel-gloved finger. Recognition that the base of the tongue falling against the posterior pharyngeal wall accounted for most airway obstruction did not occur until 1880. Credit for the first use of a true mask to deliver anesthesia is given to John Snow (1813–1858), the first real anesthesiologist. Joseph Clover used a nasopharyngeal tube for the delivery of chloroform anesthesia in 1881. The O'Dwyer tube was introduced by Joseph O'Dwyer in 1884 and consisted of a curved metal conduit with a conical end that could seal the laryngeal inlet when placed into the oropharynx. In the 1930s, Ralph Waters introduced the now-familiar flattened tube oral airway. Arthure Guedel modified Waters's concept by fitting his airway within a stiff rubber envelope in an attempt to reduce mucosal trauma.

Tracheal intubation was first described in 1788 as a means of resuscitation of the 'apparently dead,' but was not used for the delivery of anesthesia for another 100 years. The forerunner of the modern endotracheal tube was designed by the German otolaryngologist, Dr Franz Kuhn (1866–1929). Kuhn developed a flexible-metallic tube that resisted kinking and could be shaped to the patient's upper airway anatomy. It was inserted using a rigid stylet, and the hypopharynx was sealed with oiled gauze packing. Sir Ivan Magill and Stanley Rowbotham are credited with the initial development of modern visual tracheal intubation. Performing anesthesia for reconstructive facial surgery (during World War I), they developed a two-tube nasal system. One narrow tube (of a gum elastic design) was passed through the nares and guided into the larynx using a surgical laryngoscope. The other tube was blindly passed into the pharynx to allow the escape of gases. During the use of this 'Magill tube,' the exhaust lumen would occasionally pass blindly into the larynx, leading him to describe the technique as 'blind nasal intubation' (Magill 1928).

Cuffed tubes were initially described in the early part of the 20th century. Three factors led to the development of these devices:
- The introduction of cyclopropane (which was explosive and required an airtight circuit for appropriate gas containment)
- The fact that blind and laryngoscopic-guided tracheal intubation remained a difficult task
- A recognized need for protection of the lower airway from blood and surgical debris in the upper airway

The Primrose cuffed oropharyngeal tube, the Shipway airway (a Guedel oropharyngeal airway fitted with a cuff and a circuit connector designed by Sir Ivan Magill), and the Lessinger airway were predecessors of the modern supraglottic devices. In 1937, Beverley Leech introduced a 'pharyngeal bulb gasway' with a noninflatable cuff that fitted snuggly into the hypopharynx.

The use of supraglottic airways remained dominant until the introduction of curare in 1942, and the mass training of anesthesiologists in tracheal intubation in anticipation of casualties during World War II. The description by C.L. Mendelson (1946) of gastric contents aspiration in obstetric cases (66 of 44,016 patients, with 2 deaths) further pushed the move toward tracheal intubation in most surgical procedures. Within a few years, proficiency in direct laryngoscopy and tracheal intubation became a mark of professionalism. The advent of succinylcholine in 1951 furthered the dominance of tracheal intubation by providing rapid and profound muscle relaxation.

By 1981, two types of airway management prevailed: tracheal intubation or the anesthesia facemask, and each had its own failings. These difficulties led to the reconsideration of supraglottic airways and the birth of the laryngeal mask.

Perhaps the newest innovation is a distal chip video camera placed on the end of a disposable plastic laryngoscope: the GlideScope (Verathon Inc., Bothell, MA, USA) is the most successful of these (Aziz et al. 2011).

References

Aziz MF, Healy D, Kheterpal S, et al. Routine clinical practice effectiveness of the Glidescope in difficult airway management: an analysis of 2,004 Glidescope intubations, complications, and failures from two institutions. Anesthesiology 2011; 114:34–41.

Jackson CL. Tracheotomy. Laryngoscope 1909; 19:285–290.

Jones WHS. Hippocrates in English. The Classical Review 2009; 2:88–89.

Magill IW. Technique in endotracheal anesthesia. Proc Roy Soc Med 1928; 22:83–84.

Mendelson CL. The aspiration of stomach contents into the lungs during obstetric anesthesia. Am J Ostet Gynecol 1946; 52:191-205.

Stock CR. What is past is prologue: a short history of the development of tracheostomy. Ear Nose Throat J 1987; 4:166–169.

Further reading

Baker AB. Artificial respiration, the history of an idea. Medical History 1971 15; 4:336–351.

Olszewski J, Milonski J. History of tracheotomy. Otolaryngol Pol 2007; 61:349–352.

Trubuhovich RV. 19th century pioneering of intensive therapy in North America. Part 3: the Fell-O'Dwyer apparatus and William P Northrup. Crit Care Resusc 2009; 11:78–86.

Watcha MF, Garner FT, White PF, et al. Laryngeal mask vs. facemask and Gudel airway during pediatric myringotomy. Arch Otolaryngol Head Neck Surg 1994; 120:877–880.

2

Surgical anatomy of the airway

Jerome W Thompson, Karuna Dewan

The head

There is a significant difference in the size and configuration of the child's head versus that of an adult. The proportion of face to cranium is about 1:8 at birth, 1:5 at 7 years, and 1:2 as an adult (**Figure 2.1**). The cranium occupies a larger portion of the child's head and is disproportionately more susceptible to injury than the facial structures. Parts of the infant's membranous skull have not yet ossified and remain at the junctions of the firm bones as thin fibrous tissues called fontanelles. The firmness of these membranes can be an indicator of increased intracranial pressure, but they must not be pressed too firmly upon during positioning of the head for intubation.

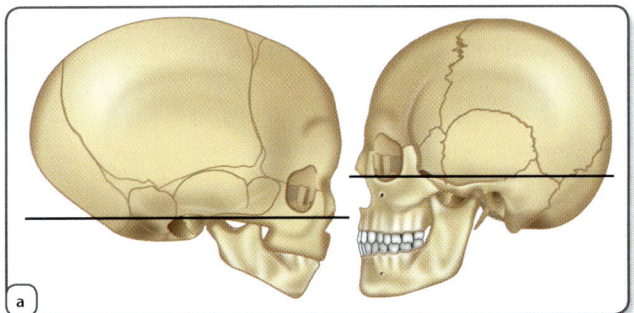

a

Figure 2.1 Head size comparison child versus adult. The horizontal rules in (a) signify the skull floor.

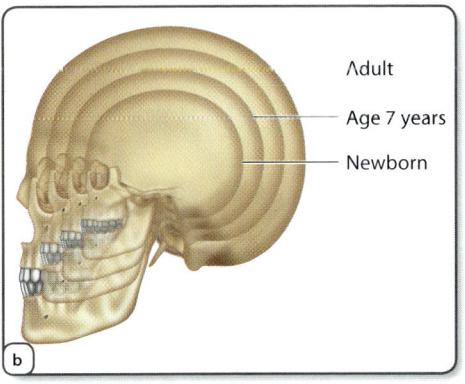

Adult

Age 7 years

Newborn

b

The nose

The external nose's internal structure is half cartilaginous, which gives it a great deal of flexibility, and half bony (and rigid). The nasal alae or anterior openings to the nose can be asymmetrical; verging on pinpoint in some cases. The limiting factor may also be the bony opening called the pyramidal aperture (**Figure 2.2**). Narrowing here, known as pyramidal aperture stenosis, can prohibit nasal intubation of either side.

Nasal cavity

The roof of the nasal cavity is made up of the cribriform plate, which is fragile and susceptible to injury in association with skull fractures, facial fractures, and surgery (Cameron & Lupton 1993). Endotracheal tubes or nasogastric tubes should not be passed through the nose if these injuries are suspected without the assistance of neurosurgical or maxillofacial surgeons. Endotracheal tubes have been accidentally passed into the brain during nasal intubation of both adult patients and infants with head trauma (**Figure 2.3**) (Krakovitz & Koltai 2010). There are three major turbinates, which act as cooling and humidification 'fins,' and which arise from the lateral wall of the interior nose. Frequently mistaken for polyps, they can undergo allergic polypoid transformations and have the appearance of an ovoid polyp, but are merely thick, membrane-covered bones. The middle turbinate bone can be flat or bulbous, containing an obstructing air-filled bony sack called a concha bullosa. These bullae can be easily fractured or compressed medially during intubation (Tanyeri et al. 2012).

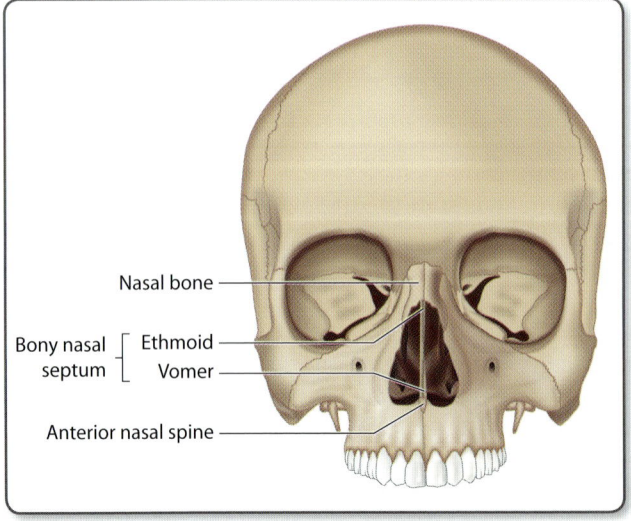

Figure 2.2 Anterior view of the nasal cavity.

Nasal bone

Bony nasal septum ⎡ Ethmoid
⎣ Vomer

Anterior nasal spine

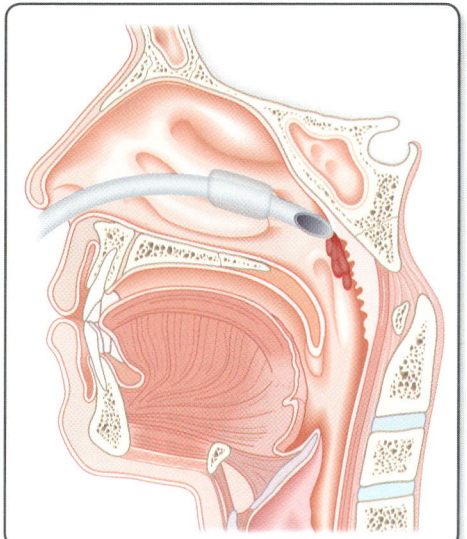

Figure 2.3 Structure of the nasal vault and endotracheal tube, showing the tube impacting the adenoid tissue.

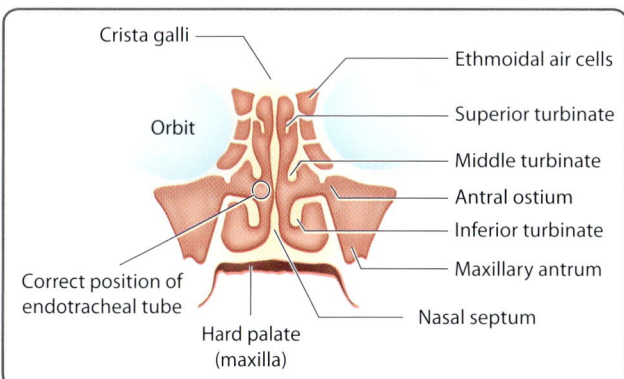

Crista galli
Orbit
Correct position of endotracheal tube
Hard palate (maxilla)
Ethmoidal air cells
Superior turbinate
Middle turbinate
Antral ostium
Inferior turbinate
Maxillary antrum
Nasal septum

Figure 2.4 View of the turbinates showing the correct positioning of the endotracheal tube.

The most likely path resulting in compression is between the inferior and the middle turbinate and sliding along the septum, since the inferior turbinate is by far the largest of the three (**Figure 2.4**). The membranes may be engorged from local allergic reactions or autonomic activity and must be shrunk with an intranasal vasoconstrictor spray prior to intubation. Lubricant must be applied to the endotracheal tube to facilitate passage through this narrow area. The mucosa is very vascular, and vasoconstricting drugs are very effective in shrinking the membranes, thus lowering resistance and allowing easier and less traumatic intubation. Epinephrine and cocaine, in combination with some anesthetic gases, have been associated with cardiac arrhythmias and arrests during nasal surgery (Richard et al. 1988).

Septum

The most common cause of airway obstruction is due to septal abnormalities. The septum is frequently distorted or deviated at birth while passing through the birth canal, and it can also be damaged later in life, secondary to trauma. This distortion can be in the form of a fracture or a severe flexion deviation. The deflection can be in the anteroposterior plane or in the cephalocaudal plane. A combination of several independent distortions or deflections can make intranasal entubation difficult, if not impossible. The nose is supplied by the sphenopalatine, palatal, anterior ethmoid, and labial arteries. A vascular structure of note is Little's area or Kiesselbach's plexus (**Figure 2.5**), in the anterior nose, which is supplied by the anterior ethmoid and labial arteries. These vessels are responsible for 90% of epistaxis cases (Kost & Post 1997), being an extremely vascular network in the anterior inferior aspect of the septum that is easily injured by a suction catheter or an endotracheal tube. To avoid injury to this plexus, the leading tip and the side holes of the endotracheal tube should be angled away from the septum and the tube should be very well lubricated. The posterior ethmoid artery completes the blood supply to the posterior nose. Bleeding from any of the above-mentioned arteries can make airway management difficult (Kucil & Clenney 2005). The choanae are the posterior openings of the nose into the nasopharynx. The floor of the nose is slightly tilted down posteriorly as compared to anteriorly, so the intubation tube should be angled down as it is inserted.

Nasopharynx

The adenoid is not a smooth rounded structure as seen in most textbooks, but rather a deeply pocketed irregular mass of lymphoid tissue. This is important, in that the pockets can entrap a flexible fiberoptic scope and break the guide-wires that steer it when in the hands of a novice.

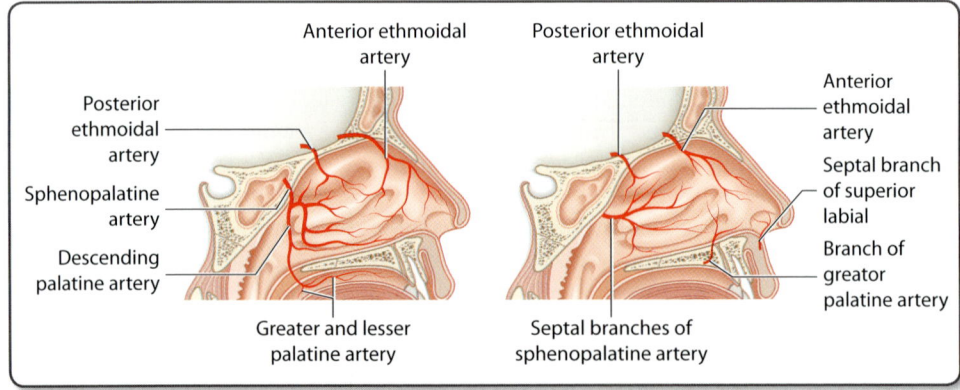

Figure 2.5 View of septal distortions and Kiesselbach's plexus.

The adenoid is soft and can be impaled by an endotracheal tube, impeding the passage of the tube and leading to profuse bleeding. They can also hypertrophy, encroach upon, and engulf the choanae, or enter into the posterior nasal cavity, completely obstructing it, and preventing the passage of fiberoptic scopes or endotracheal tubes (**Figure 2.6**).

Oral cavity

Maxilla

The upper teeth are embedded in the paired maxillary bones. These bones are stable and only mobile when there is a Le Fort I, II, or III fracture of the face. When these bones are mobile, entubation can be compromised (**Figure 2.7**).

Mandible

The location of the lower jaw or mandible can be classified in roughly one of three positions using Angle's classification of the permanent teeth (Brin et al. 2000) (**Figure 2.8**).

Normal, neutrocclusion or class I occlusion is where the first maxillary molar is slightly posterior to the first mandibular molar and

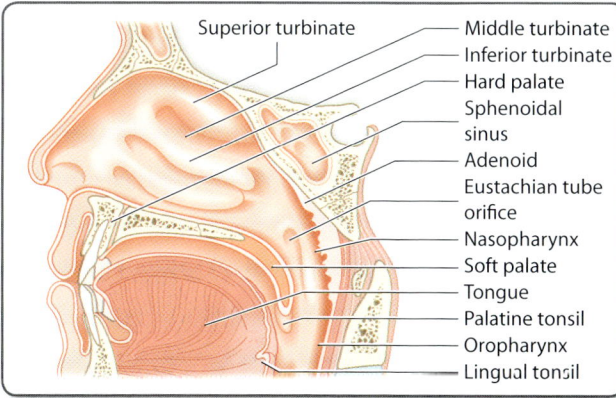

Superior turbinate — Middle turbinate
Inferior turbinate
Hard palate
Sphenoidal sinus
Adenoid
Eustachian tube orifice
Nasopharynx
Soft palate
Tongue
Palatine tonsil
Oropharynx
Lingual tonsil

Figure 2.6 View of lateral half of skull showing nasopharynx.

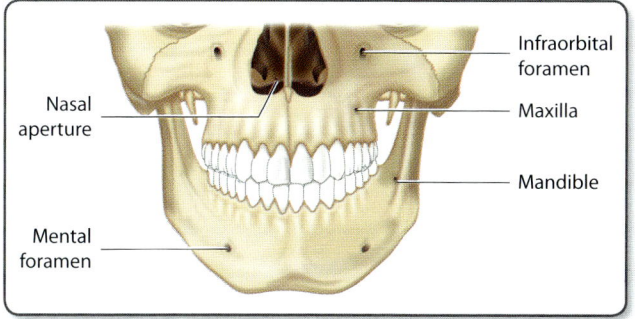

Nasal aperture
Mental foramen
Infraorbital foramen
Maxilla
Mandible

Figure 2.7 AP view of the maxilla and mandible.

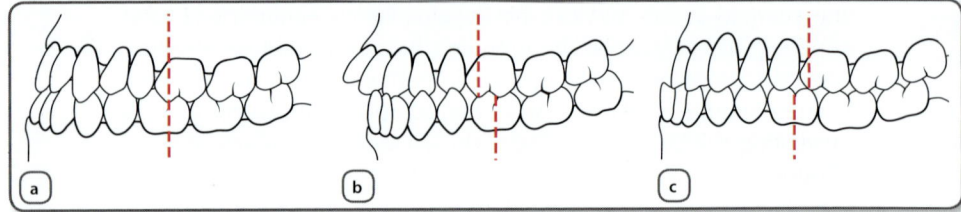

Figure 2.8 View of three mandibular occlusions: (a) normal, (b) distocclusion and (c) mesiocclusion.

the mesiobuccal or forward cusp rests in the valley or buccal groove of the first mandibular molar. Buckteeth, distocclusion, or class II occlusion is where the first maxillary molar is just forward of the mandibular molar, and the mesiobuccal or forward cusp rests anterior to the valley or buccal groove of the first mandibular molar. If the jaw is severely retrognathic, class II occlusion can be associated with a small jaw that can obstruct one's ability to be intubated orally such as in the Pierre Robin Sequence. Prognathic, mesiocclusion, or class III occlusion is where the lower jaw juts out and the mesiobuccal cusp of the first maxillary molar rests posterior to the mandibular buccal groove. The temporomandibular joint is a complex joint with four articular surfaces that give it multidirectional capabilities.

Tongue

Embryologically, the tongue arises from two separate anlage: anterior and posterior. If the front half fails to form normally, the jaw will be excessively narrow and again present difficulties with intubation. The base of the tongue faces the oropharynx and is covered with the lingual tonsils, which can become hypertrophic (**Figure 2.9**). These can obstruct the airway and need to be surgically debulked. There are syndromes where the tongue is excessively large as in Beckwith–Wiedemann syndrome, hemangiomas, hamartomas, and lymphangioimas. These patients

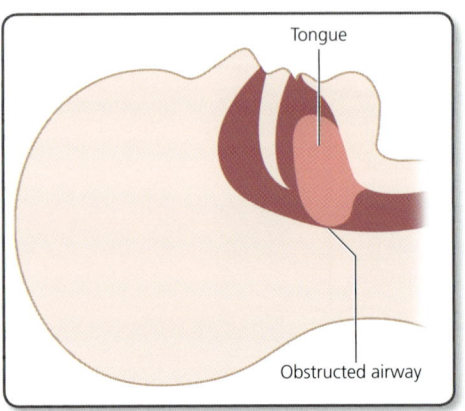

Tongue

Obstructed airway

Figure 2.9 Tongue obstruction in an unconscious patient.

may require a tracheotomy in order to be ventilated (Farrell 1995). The Mallampati scale evaluates the degree of epiglottic visibility over the tongue and therefore the ease or difficulty of intubation (Mallampati et al. 1985) (**Figure 2.10**). The lingual nerve innervates the anterior two-thirds of the tongue. The glossopharyngeal nerve innervates the posterior one-third of the tongue, including the circumvallate papillae. Taste fibers in the lingual nerve originate from the geniculate ganglion of the facial nerve and join the lingual nerve via the chorda tympani. The vallecula was called the 'diamond smuggler's pouch' because diamonds could be held undetected there for long periods of time. Food, foreign bodies, and pills can also catch there. It is in this pouch that the distal tip of the Macintosh laryngoscope blade is placed, at the junction of the epiglottis and the posterior base of the tongue.

Hypopharynx

In the second year of life, the larynx descends in the neck. This is associated with pharyngeal elongation. As a result, the soft palate and the larynx are no longer in contact but are separated by a significant gap. The gap is essentially a growth of the hypopharyngeal space. This allows for greater vocal power and diversity in sound generation or articulation. This growth and separation increases the complexity of the swallowing process. The epiglottis and the uvula are no longer in contact. The laryngopharynx extends superiorly from the level of the hyoid bone down to the lower border of the cricoid cartilage (**Figure 2.11**). It tapers narrowly at the upper end of the esophagus. The posterior border is the hyoid bone and thyroid cartilage. Anteriorly, the larynx, the epiglottis, and the arytenoids delineate the laryngopharynx.

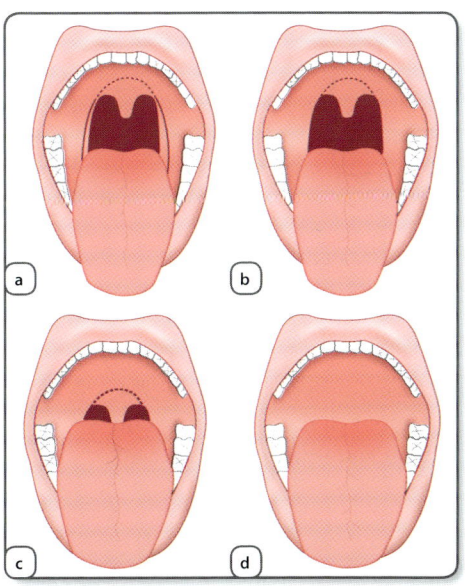

Figure 2.10 Mallampati scale. (a) Class I: soft palate, uvula, fauces, pillars visible – no difficulty with intubation. (b) Class II: soft palate, uvula, fauces visible – no difficulty with intubation. (c) Class III: soft palate, base of uvula visible – moderate difficulty with intubation. (d) Class IV: hard palate only visible – severe difficulty with intubation.

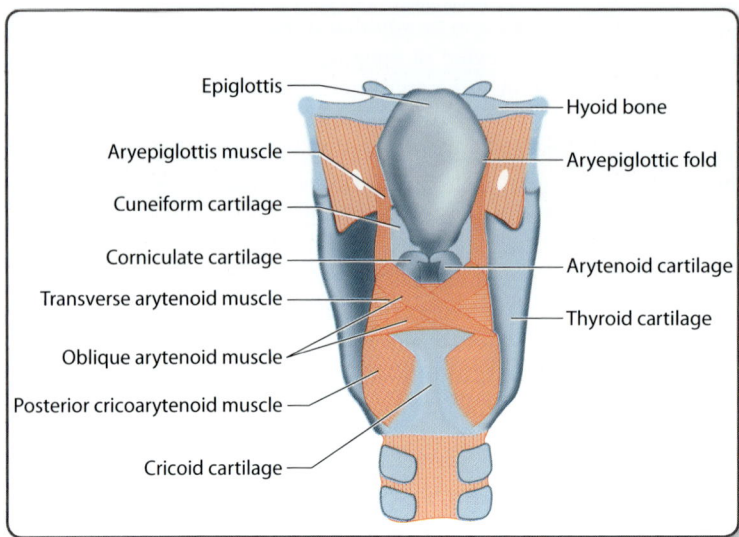

Figure 2.11 Posterior view of the larynx/pharynx.

Epiglottis

Aryepiglottis muscle

Cuneiform cartilage

Corniculate cartilage

Transverse arytenoid muscle

Oblique arytenoid muscle

Posterior cricoarytenoid muscle

Cricoid cartilage

Hyoid bone

Aryepiglottic fold

Arytenoid cartilage

Thyroid cartilage

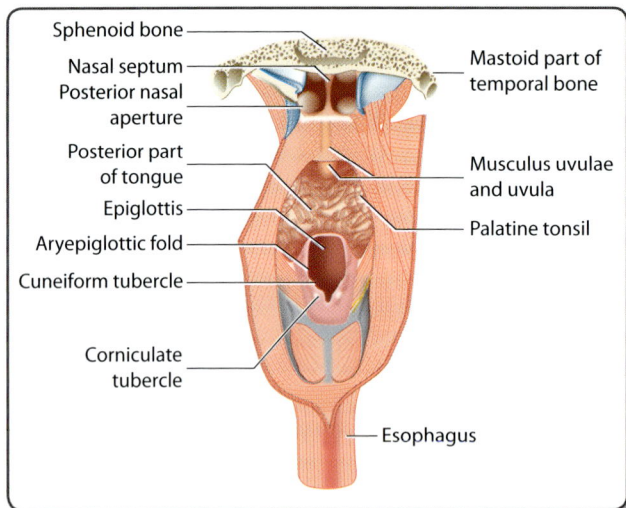

Figure 2.12 Pyriform fossa.

Sphenoid bone

Nasal septum

Posterior nasal aperture

Posterior part of tongue

Epiglottis

Aryepiglottic fold

Cuneiform tubercle

Corniculate tubercle

Mastoid part of temporal bone

Musculus uvulae and uvula

Palatine tonsil

Esophagus

The hyoid bone is the bony structure that is the foundation for the tongue muscles. It is also the point of most effective anterior pressure to visualize the larynx during intubation. Since it is easily palpated, it can be mistaken for the cricoid cartilage, and a cricothyrotomy can therefore be placed too high above the larynx, with disastrous results. The pyriform fossae are funnel-shaped regions of the distal throat on either side of the larynx that can direct errant endotracheal tubes easily into the upper esophagus (**Figure 2.12**).

Laryngeal complex

The laryngeal skeleton is made of one bone and several cartilages strung together in series and suspended from the skull base and mandible (**Figure 2.13**). Laryngeal motion is caused by intrinsic muscle action as well as the action of the extrinsic muscles. The hyoid, which supports the larynx and stabilizes the hypopharynx, is U-shaped and is connected to the thyroid cartilage by the broad thyrohyoid membrane. The thyroid cartilage is composed of two halves fused anteriorly at a sharp angle. The superior cornu of the thyroid cartilage attaches to the thyrohyoid ligament, whereas the inferior cornu articulates with the cricoid cartilage. The epiglottis is a fibroelastic cartilage, attached (anteriorly to the midline) to the inner surface of the thyroid cartilage and supported by the hyoepiglottic ligament. The cricoid cartilage supplies skeletal support to the subglottis. The subglottis is the only

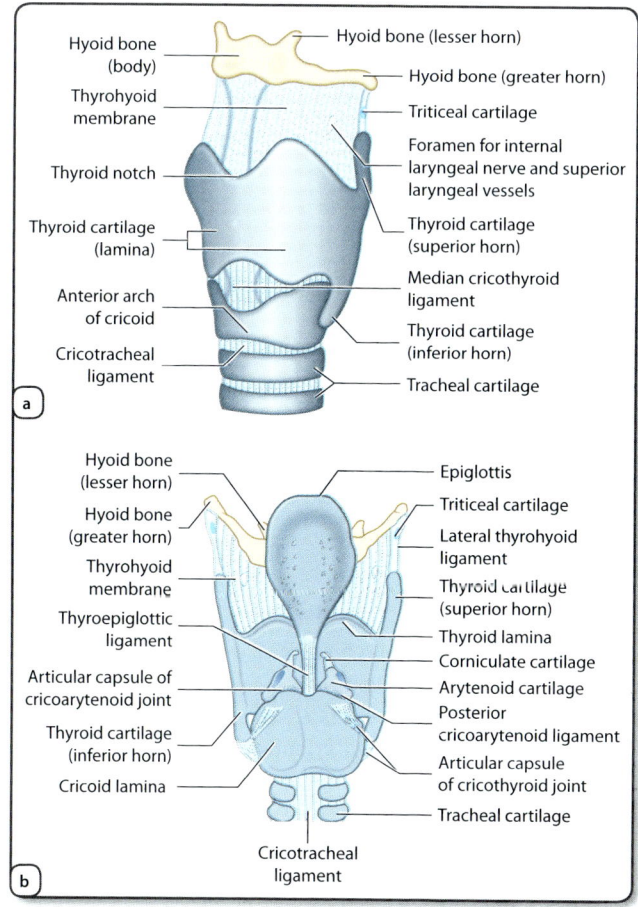

Figure 2.13 Hyolaryngeal skeleton.

a

Hyoid bone (body)
Thyrohyoid membrane
Thyroid notch
Thyroid cartilage (lamina)
Anterior arch of cricoid
Cricotracheal ligament

Hyoid bone (lesser horn)
Hyoid bone (greater horn)
Triticeal cartilage
Foramen for internal laryngeal nerve and superior laryngeal vessels
Thyroid cartilage (superior horn)
Median cricothyroid ligament
Thyroid cartilage (inferior horn)
Tracheal cartilage

b

Hyoid bone (lesser horn)
Hyoid bone (greater horn)
Thyrohyoid membrane
Thyroepiglottic ligament
Articular capsule of cricoarytenoid joint
Thyroid cartilage (inferior horn)
Cricoid lamina

Epiglottis
Triticeal cartilage
Lateral thyrohyoid ligament
Thyroid cartilage (superior horn)
Thyroid lamina
Corniculate cartilage
Arytenoid cartilage
Posterior cricoarytenoid ligament
Articular capsule of cricothyroid joint
Tracheal cartilage

Cricotracheal ligament

portion of the airway with a completely rigid circular structure (**Figure 2.14**). It has a smaller cross-sectional area than the trachea. Anteriorly, the cricoid is 1 cm high, with a smooth, curved surface. Posteriorly, it is 2–3 cm high and the superior surface is flattened centrally to provide an area of articulation for the arytenoid cartilages. Posterolaterally, on each side, the cricoid articulates with the inferior cornu of the thyroid cartilage, allowing rotation in a sagittal plane, opening and closing the anterior cricothyroid space. Each arytenoid cartilage is pear-shaped. The broad base articulates with the cricoid in a synovial joint, allowing movement in multiple axes. The vocal process, the anterior and medial projection of the arytenoid, is the posterior segment emanating from the membranous vocal fold (**Figure 2.15**). Two other small sesamoid cartilages, the corniculate and the cuneiform, are located superior to the arytenoid and support the aryepiglottic fold. The conus elasticus is a fibroelastic membrane that provides support to the vocal fold. The quadrangular membrane similarly supports the supraglottis, connecting the epiglottis to the arytenoid. The superior edge forms the aryepiglottic fold, while the intrinsic laryngeal muscles are primarily responsible for the motion of the vocal folds. The posterior cricoarytenoid muscle is the only abductor of the glottis and originates from the posterior surface of the cricoid, inserting onto the muscular process of the arytenoid. The lateral cricoarytenoid muscle

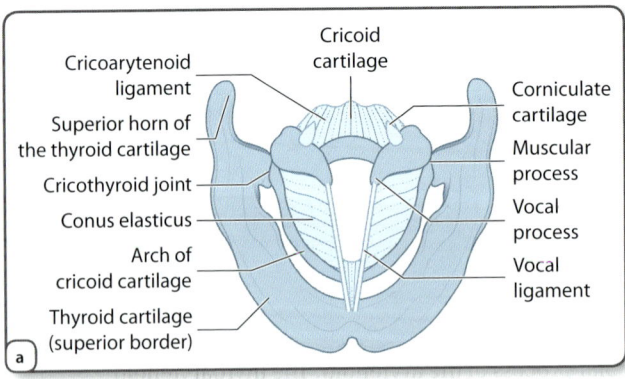

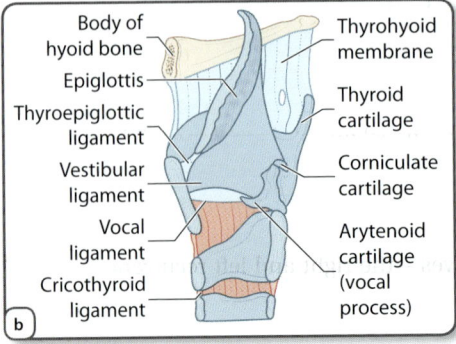

Figure 2.14 (a) Anteroposterior cricoids and (b) lateral cricoid.

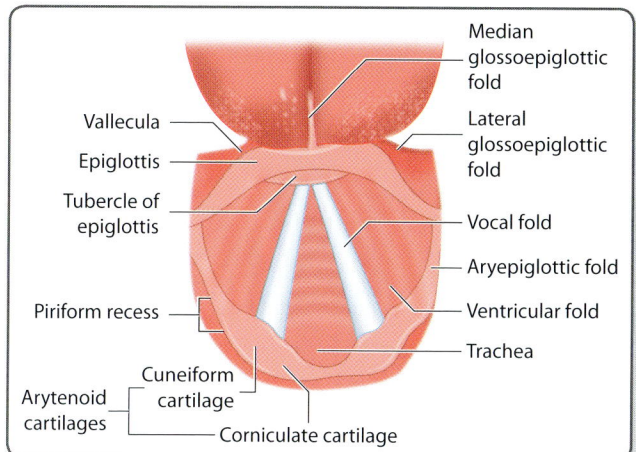

Figure 2.15 Vocal cord anatomy.

Median glossoepiglottic fold

Lateral glossoepiglottic fold

Vallecula

Epiglottis

Tubercle of epiglottis

Vocal fold

Aryepiglottic fold

Piriform recess

Ventricular fold

Trachea

Cuneiform cartilage

Arytenoid cartilages

Corniculate cartilage

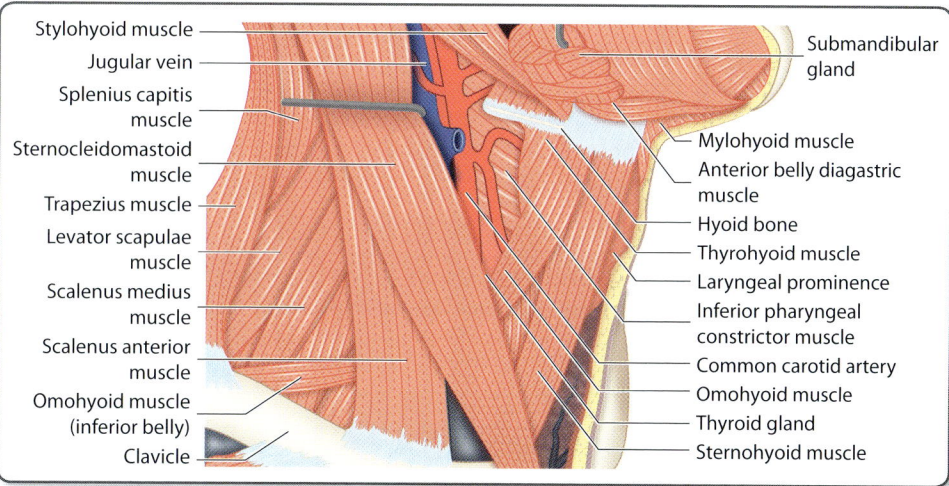

Figure 2.16 Muscles of the lateral neck with bony landmarks.

Stylohyoid muscle

Jugular vein

Splenius capitis muscle

Sternocleidomastoid muscle

Trapezius muscle

Levator scapulae muscle

Scalenus medius muscle

Scalenus anterior muscle

Omohyoid muscle (inferior belly)

Clavicle

Submandibular gland

Mylohyoid muscle

Anterior belly diagastric muscle

Hyoid bone

Thyrohyoid muscle

Laryngeal prominence

Inferior pharyngeal constrictor muscle

Common carotid artery

Omohyoid muscle

Thyroid gland

Sternohyoid muscle

is an adductor with its origin on the lateral aspect of the cricoid and insertion on the muscular process of the arytenoid. The thyroarytenoid muscle arises from the inner aspect of the thyroid cartilage and inserts on the vocal process of the arytenoid. Contraction of this muscle results in increasing vocal fold tension, thickness, and stiffness. The only unpaired laryngeal muscle is the interarytenoid, the function of which is to adduct the vocal folds. Extrinsic laryngeal muscles are responsible for elevating or depressing the larynx or moving it in the anteroposterior plane. They include the mylohyoid, digastric, stylohyoid, omohyoid, sternohyoid, sternothyroid, and thyrohyoid (**Figure 2.16**). The larynx is supplied by two paired sets of nerves – the right and left recurrent motor nerves and the right and left superior laryngeal sensory nerves (**Figure 2.17**).

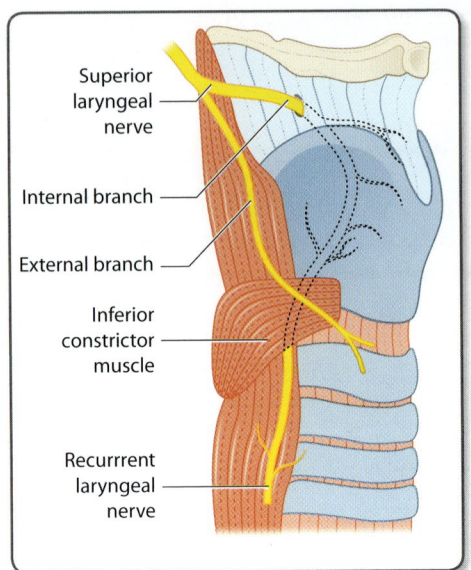

Figure 2.17 Laryngeal nerves.

Superior laryngeal nerve

Internal branch

External branch

Inferior constrictor muscle

Recurrrent laryngeal nerve

The neck

Cervical spine

C1–C2 subluxation is a risk in children with Down syndrome (Selby et al. 1991) (**Figure 2.18**). Deep neck spaces are embryologic spaces that contain the spread of neck infection. They have discrete fascial layers, which typically limit infection to the neck and away from the chest

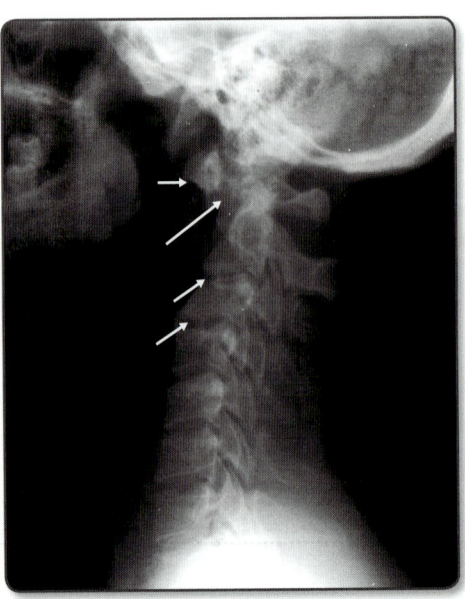

Figure 2.18 Vertebral subluxation X-ray image. With permission from Ali FE, Al-Bustan MA, Al-Busairi WA, et al. Cervical spine abnormalities associated with Down syndrome. Int Orthop 2006; 30:284-289.

and mediastinum. The vascular sheath, though, extends from the skull to the heart and can thus act as a conduit for infection (**Figure 2.19**). The retropharyngeal space also can act as a pathway for infection to spread from the skull base through the retroperitoneum to the coccyx. A retropharyngeal abscess can be so large as to obstruct the airway by pressing onto the larynx, presenting a difficult intubation, or worse still, rupturing during intubation. There are three major deep neck spaces of concern: the retropharyngeal, danger, and prevertebral space. Infections here can spread from the skull base, via the mediastinum, to the coccyx.

The carotid and the jugular veins are at risk during neck surgery due to the hyperextension of the neck required to expose other structures such as the trachea. Usually, this maneuver pushes the trachea up anteriorly, but sometimes the great vessels are equally prominent. In emergent slash tracheotomies, the incision should be vertical to avoid these vessels (**Figure 2.20**).

Esophagus

The entrotus or upper opening of the esophagus is just behind the larynx and has the cricoid as its anterior wall. It is only a potential space but is larger than the laryngeal vocal cord opening, so it can more easily be intubated than the larynx (Reyes et al. 1992) (**Figure 2.21**).

Trachea

Embryologically, the trachea, as with the larynx, formed a solid tube that hollowed out, thus explaining many unfortunate abnormalities. It connects to the cricoid cartilage and travels into the chest to the bronchi (**Figure 2.21**). The cartilages are U-shaped, with thin membranes connecting them like pearls on a necklace.

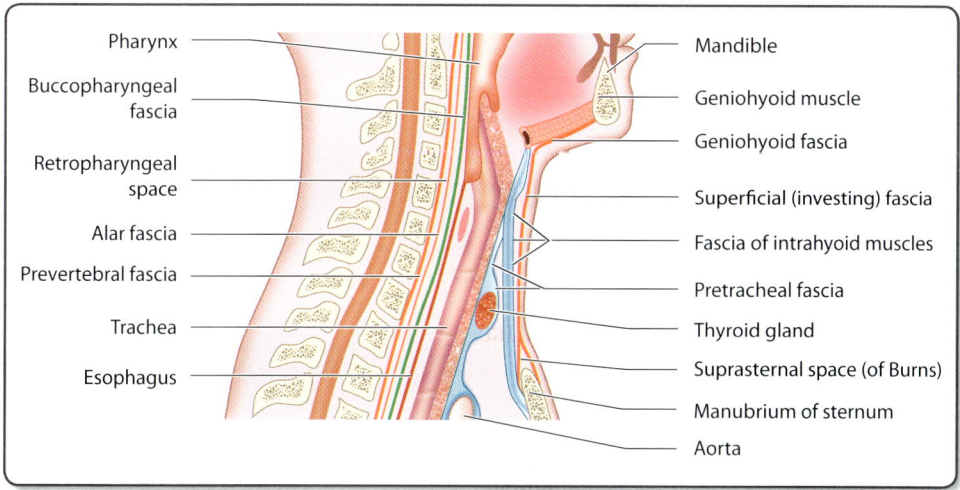

Figure 2.19 Neck spaces.

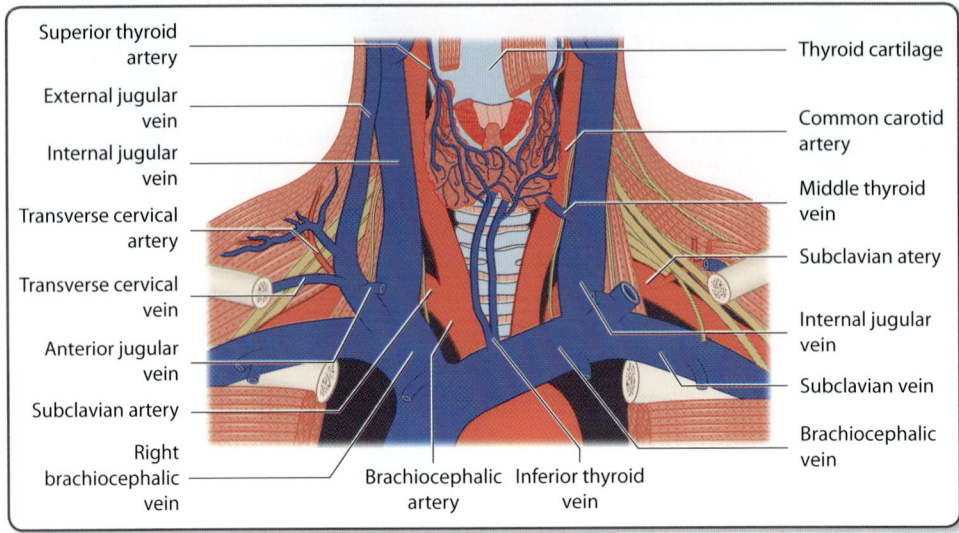

Figure 2.20 Major neck vasculature and vascular supply to the thyroid, demonstrating the danger of neck exploration for airway trauma and tracheotomy.

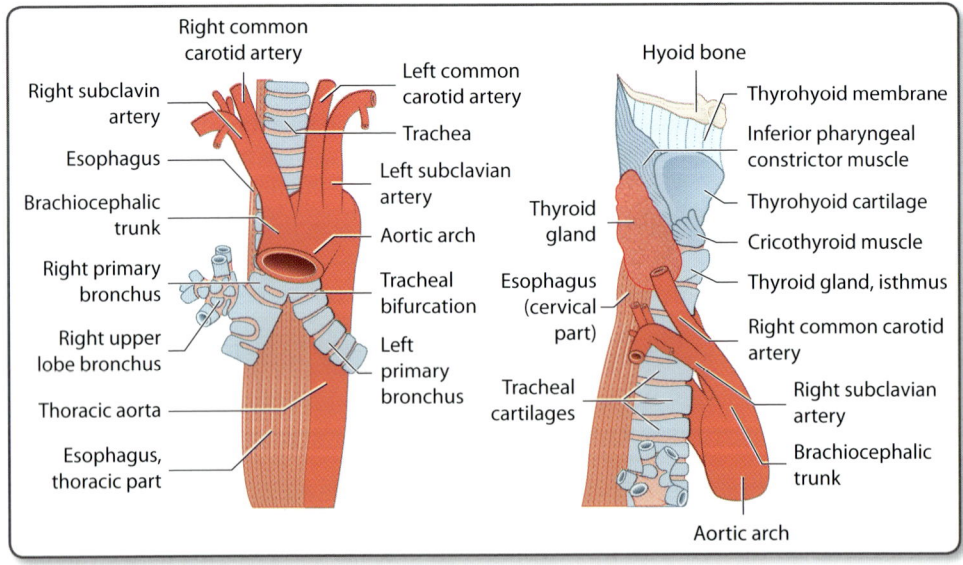

Figure 2.21 Esophagus and trachea: (a) Anteroposterior and (b) lateral views. These views show the close relationship of the airway to the aorta and esophagus which are frequently injured simultaneously.

Thyroid

The thyroid is a large endocrine structure on the anterior tracheal wall and is frequently an obstacle to a tracheotomy. It is located just below the cricoid and above the sternal notch and has significant bilateral, superior, and inferior blood supply. In the embryo, it descends into the neck from the level of the tongue so that several anatomic abnormalities can arise at different levels (**Figure 2.21**).

Conclusion

A detailed knowledge of the neck vascular muscular and organ structure is essential for the management of the airway, especially with trauma and tracheostomy.

References

Brin I, Weinberger T, Ben-Chorin E. Classification of occlusion reconsidered. Eur Orthod 2000; 22:169–174.

Cameron D, Lupton BA. Inadvertent brain penetration during neonatal nasotracheal intubation. Arch Dis Child 1993; 69:79–80.

Farrell RW. Tracheostomy may not be necessary during surgery. BJM 1995; 4:329.

Krakovitz PR, Koltai PJ. Pediatric facial fractures. In: Flint PW, Haughey BH, Lund LJ, et al. (eds), Cummings otolaryngology: head and neck surgery, 5th edn. Philadelphia: Mosby, 2010: chapter 189.

Kost SI, Post CJ. Management of epistaxis. In: Henretic FM, King C (eds), Textbook of pediatric emergency procedures. Baltimore: Lippincott Williams and Wilkins, 1997:664: chapter 60.

Kucil CJ, Clenney T. Management of epistaxis. Am Fam Physician 2005; 71:305–311.

Mallampati SR, Gatt SP, Gugino LD, et al. A clinical sign to predict difficult intubation: a prospective study. Can Anaesth Soc J 1985; 32: 429–434.

Reyes G, Galvis AG, Thompson JW. Esophageal perforation during an emergency intubation. Am J Emerg Med 1992; 10:223–225.

Richard W, Thompson JW, Lewis G, Levy DS, Church JA. Cardiac arrest with halothane anesthesia in a patient receiving theophylline. Ann Allergy 1988; 61:83–84.

Selby KA, Newton RW, Gupta S, Hunt L. Clinical predictors and radiological reliability in atlantoaxial subluxation in Down's syndrome. Arch Dis Child 1991; 66:876–878.

Tanyeri H, Aksoy EA, Serin GM, et al. Will a crushed concha bullosa form again? Laryngoscope 2012; 122:956–960.

Further reading

Clemente CD. Anatomy: a regional atlas of the human body, 6th edn. Philadelphia: Lippincott Williams and Wilkins, 2010.

King C, Henretic FM. Textbook of pediatric emergency procedures, 2nd edn. Philadelphia: Lippincott Williams and Wilkins, 2007.

Koehntop DE, Liao JC, Van Bergen FH. Effects if pharmacologic alterations of adrenergic mechanisms by cocaine, tropolone, aminophylline, and ketamine on epinephrine-induced arrhythmias during halothanenitrous oxide anesthesia. Anesthesiology 1977; 46:83–93

Walls RM, Murphy MF. Manual of emergency airway management, 4th edn. Philadelphia: Lippincott Williams and Wilkins, 2012.

3

Imaging the airway

Sridhar Shankar, R Ian Gray

Introduction

Airway imaging has significantly advanced since the Egyptians of 3600 BC. After millennia of direct visualization, illustrations, and pathologic analysis, Wilhelm Roentgen discovered X-rays in 1895. By 1896, the medical potential of these mysterious r ays had been realized, and the field of radiology was born. Over the next 120 years, medical imaging has revolutionized surgical planning, ensuring that surgical intervention has all available knowledge at hand, minimizing patient risk and maximizing surgical success.

Imaging techniques

Medical imaging employs advanced diagnostic techniques that supplement direct visualization and endoscopic evaluations. Each technique offers a unique viewpoint of the patient's anatomy, physiology, and pathology. Furthermore, each technique offers some advantages and disadvantages, including considerations of cost, radiation exposure, and limitations of the modality itself. The order of appropriateness of a particular modality depends largely on what is available in any given setting. Sonography is the most portable and affordable technique, providing excellent visualization of the structures around the airway, allowing rapid analysis of the vasculature prior to or during intervention, but it is limited in its assessment of the airway itself. Radiographs and fluoroscopy are more available in outpatient or rural settings. Furthermore, computed tomography (CT) is the best modality for the rapid analysis of complex pathology. Understanding the acuity needed in airway management, as well as underlying pathology, will allow for an appropriate imaging approach in both the acute and ongoing settings.

Radiography

Radiography is a fast, affordable, and relatively low-radiation modality, best used for initial assessment in conjunction with the findings of a physical examination. Five main densities are visible: air, fat, soft tissue or fluid, calcium, and radiodense foreign matter. While the limited contrast resolution prevents detailed demonstration of the underlying anatomy, the unparalleled spatial resolution creates an irreplaceable 'roadmap' for initial assessment and surgical planning.

Nasopharyngeal airway assessment

The traditional radiographic analysis of the nasopharyngeal airway may include a Water's view (angled through the chin with the patient's head tilted up), a Caldwell's view [straight anteroposterior (AP)], a Towne's view (looking down), a lateral view, and potentially oblique mandibular views (**Figures 3.1** and **3.2**). The lateral view is the most informative, including visualization of the nasal airway, uvula, adenoids, hard palate, mandible, and craniocervical junction. Any deviation in these structures may impair normal respiration or increase the risks of airway placement, particularly in the setting of trauma. The Caldwell's view allows for characterization of the nasal septum and airway, potentially guiding nasal cannula placement. The remaining views are most informative for off-midline pathology or trauma. In the emergent setting, radiographs provide a fast and easy assessment of mandibular, cervical, and skull base integrity; compromise to any of which may increase the risks of airway placement.

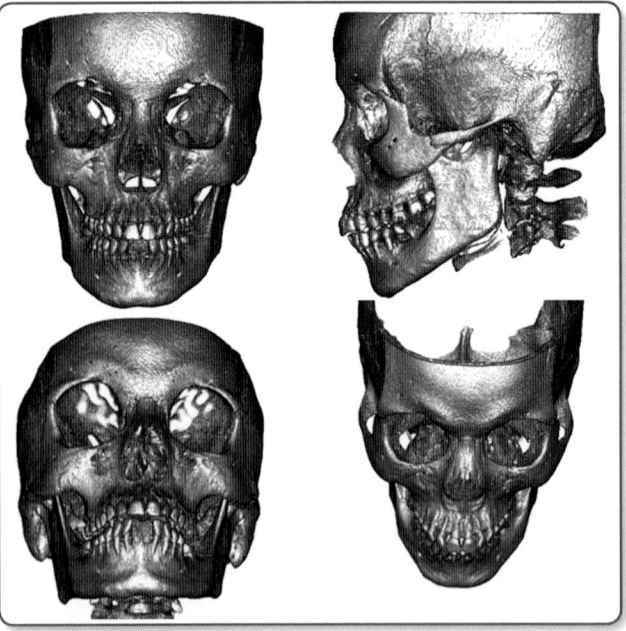

Figure 3.1 Traditional radiographic views. Clockwise from top left: Caldwell's, Lateral, Towne's, and Water's views.

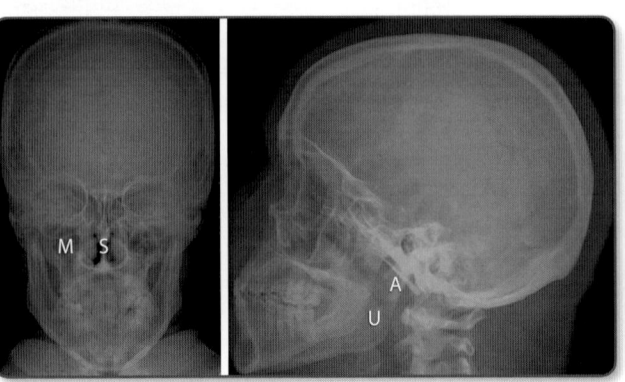

Figure 3.2 Anteroposterior (AP) and lateral facial radiographs. AP images (Caldwell's view) provide good visualization of the nasal airway and septum. The lateral view, in contrast, provides good visualization of the expected pharyngeal anatomy. A, adenoids; M, maxillary sinus; S, nasal septum; U, uvula.

Cervical airway assessment

While there are subtle differences in technique between the cervical spine analysis and the soft tissue neck analysis, the overlap often provides adequate visualization of the pertinent structures for airway assessment and planning. The core images begin with the AP and lateral neck images, with additional odontoid imaging if there is concern for instability or trauma in that region (**Figure 3.3**). The most informative view is the lateral view, which provides good visualization of the airway (including the nasopharynx, epiglottis, vestibule, glottis, and cervical trachea), prevertebral soft tissues, and cervical spine (**Figure 3.4**). A lateral view will quickly differentiate between endotracheal and esophageal localization of support devices. Prevertebral soft tissue thickening may provide the only clue to ligamentous injury in unstable cervical spine trauma. Finally, it is vital to recognize traumatic subluxation prior to aggressive cervical manipulation. The AP view provides a 'second look' of the airway, particularly visualizing any off mid-line defects.

Fluoroscopy

Fluoroscopy, or its alternative appellation, image intensifier TV (IITV) is the real-time evaluation of the anatomy and physiology of the patient utilizing a video feed of radiographic imaging. As such, it can significantly increase the radiation dose, depending on the skill of the user. It provides excellent characterization of a patient's normal functions, provides utility in intraoperative assessment and

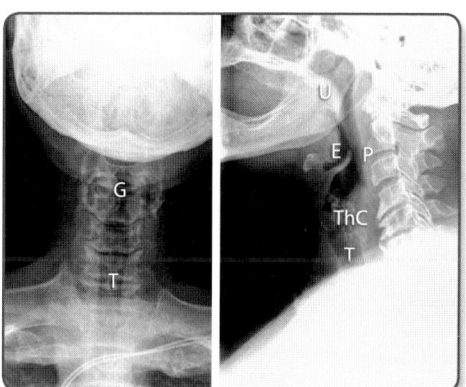

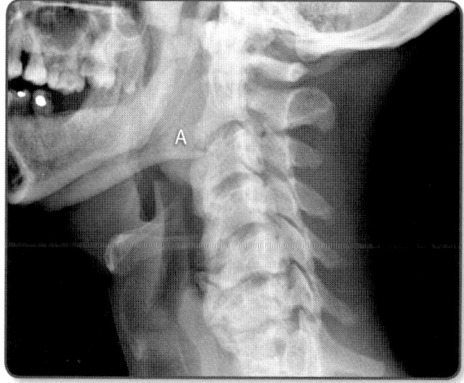

Figure 3.3 Anteroposterior (AP) and lateral neck radiographs. AP images provide good visualization of the laryngeal ventricle and subglottic airway, while the lateral view demonstrates a more optimal pharyngeal evaluation. Note that it is relatively common for heterogeneous thyroid cartilage calcification to degrade visualization of the glottis. E, epiglottis; P, prevertebral soft tissues; ThC, thyroid cartilage (heterogeneously calcified); T, trachea; U, uvula.

Figure 3.4 Improved airway visualization. In this case, direct laryngeal visualization was largely obscured by a prevertebral mass (A, abscess), but the radiograph shows the inferior extent of the lesion and good aeration of the distal airway.

guidance, and visualization of occult lesions only visible during physiologic procedures (such as breathing, swallowing, coughing, and the Valsalva maneuver). Apart from the intraoperative setting, its greatest utility in airway assessment is in the use of barium to allow the visualization of motor dysfunction, fistula or diverticula formation that may increase the risk for aspiration or impair normal respiration (**Figure 3.5**).

Computed tomography

Computed tomography (CT) utilizes a focused X-ray beam spun around the patient to create an image. The relative radiation dose is significantly higher than with plain radiography, but still within normal safety parameters if used sparingly. The additional costs include significantly increased radiation dose to the patient and financial costs to the healthcare system. The benefit is that CT yields better visualization of pathology than is invisible on plain film. A CT image can be optimized for osseous evaluation, soft tissue characterization, vascular analysis, or depiction of inflammatory and neoplastic processes. Achieving the highest diagnostic yield necessitates 'asking a specific question.' This allows for image optimization, radiation and contrast dose adjustment, and provides limited characterization of extraneous structures. Plain CT (with no intravenous contrast) evaluation is best utilized for characterizing bony injury or in patients for whom intravenous contrast is contraindicated (**Figure 3.6**). Intravenous contrast-enhanced CT (CECT) examinations can be performed in the early arterial phase to assess vascular anatomy or injury, or in a delayed phase, increasing the sensitivity for infectious or neoplastic processes (**Figure 3.7**). Furthermore, postprocessing techniques are increasingly employed to recreate surgical views, as in virtual laryngoscopy (**Figure 3.7a**) or to highlight the structure of interest and downplay peripheral distractions on the cross-sectional images (**Figure 3.7b, c**).

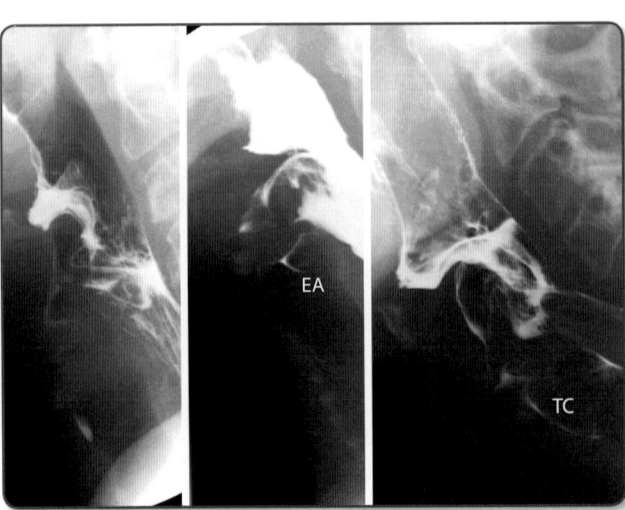

Figure 3.5 Fluoroscopy. While barium bronchograms are no longer commonplace, swallowing examinations may easily illustrate functional pathology predisposing a patient to aspiration. In this case, sequential images, from left to right, show laryngeal penetration and aspiration of barium, coating the trachea and confirming a continued risk to the airway. EA, early aspiration; TC, tracheal coating.

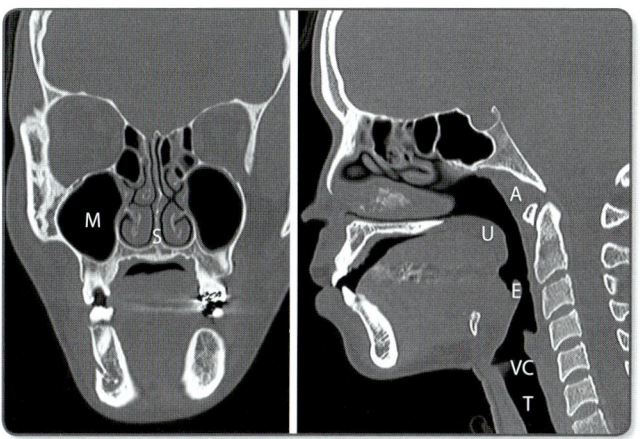

Figure 3.6 Computed tomography (CT) of the pharyngeal airway. CT is acquired as axial images that can be reconstructed in any plane. These images attempt to recreate the traditional radiographic views with improved imaging of the underlying anatomy. Patient positioning (scan angle, open mouth, or puffed cheek) can be optimized for oral evaluation if needed. A, adenoids; E, epiglottis; M, maxillary sinus; S, nasal septum; T, trachea; U, uvula; VC, vocal cords.

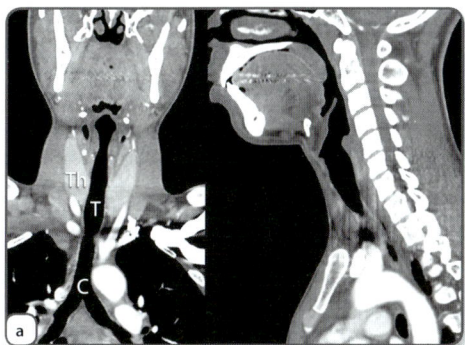

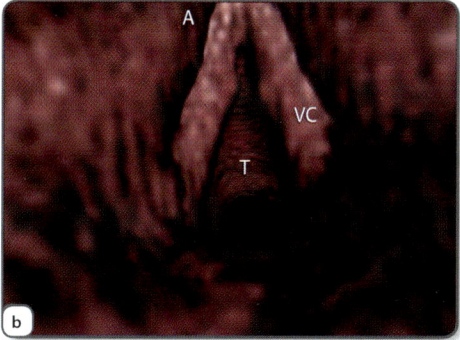

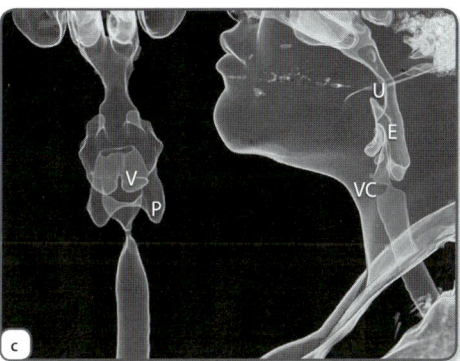

Figure 3.7 (a) Computed tomography (CT) of the cervical airway. Sample image selection reproduces the cervical radiographs, providing improved characterization of the airway and peripheral structures. C, carina; T, trachea; Th, thyroid. (b) Virtual laryngoscopy. Created with open-source software (Osirix), CT data can be reconstructed to create fly-throughs and virtual laryngoscopies in real-time for those more familiar with direct visualization. This increases patient comfort over direct laryngoscopy but diminishes sensitivity for sessile pathology. T, trachea; VC, vocal cord. (c) 3D postprocessing. Created with proprietary software (Carestream), CT data can be reconstructed for virtually any purpose. In this case, there is exquisite visualization of the airway that would increase the ease of assessing a significant deformity. E, epiglottis; P, pyriform sinus; U, uvula; V, vallecula; VC, vocal cords.

Magnetic resonance imaging

Magnetic resonance imaging (MRI) may have limited utility in visualizing the airway or in airway management in the acute setting, but it provides unparalleled soft tissue characterization without ionizing radiation (**Figure 3.8**). Despite the absence of ionizing radiation, MRI has its own significant risks, particularly with the increased prevalence of implantable medical devices. It uses high-strength magnets to exploit the electromagnetic properties of hydrogen—plentiful in tissues—to provide an image. In doing so, it deposits electromagnetic energy into the patient. As a result, the potential risks include ballistic injury, heating, and torque, each potentially life-threatening if not addressed. Once a patient is cleared of dangerous implants, MRI may provide increased specificity on the resectability of certain tumors, allowing for improved preoperative planning. One caveat is that not all MRI images are created equally. Developing a rapport with the imaging department will provide improved results, as those institutions that evaluate the most neck examinations will have the best equipment and scanning protocols.

Ultrasonography

Sonography is portable, affordable, and nearly ubiquitous, making it a good candidate for early assessment of the neck. However, ultrasound waves cannot penetrate tissue/air interfaces or hard structures such as bone, so sonography cannot image air-filled structures or tissues deep to calcifications or bone. While the airway itself is poorly visualized, its superficial nature allows for exquisite visualization of the paratracheal tissues (**Figure 3.9**). Potential utility includes the assessment of superficial vessels or the thyroid prior to percutaneous tracheostomy and characterization of infectious or soft tissue processes that may compromise the airway. While there is a theoretical risk of heating, this proves inconsequential in the normal diagnostic setting, making this the safest imaging modality available. The only real risk is not seeing the pathology of interest, which is why the expertise of the sonographer is paramount.

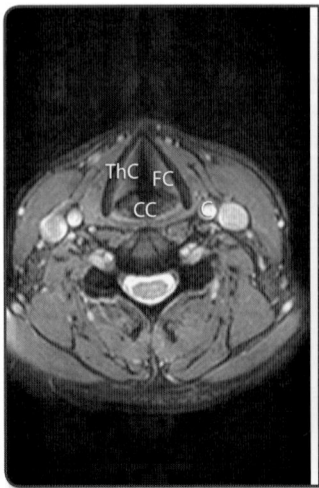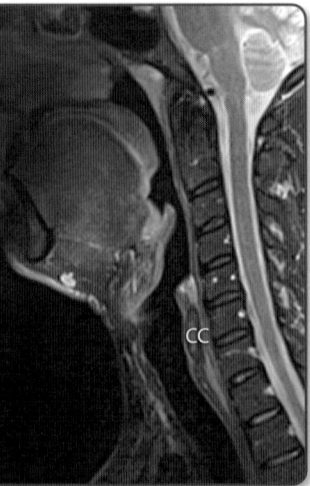

Figure 3.8 Magnetic resonance imaging (MRI) of the cervical airway. While not useful in the acute setting, preoperative planning in the setting of malignancy often relies on the improved soft tissue characterization of MRI to predict resectability and guide management. In this case, there is exquisite visualization of the larynx in a normal patient. CC, cricoid cartilage; FC, false cord; ThC, thyroid cartilage.

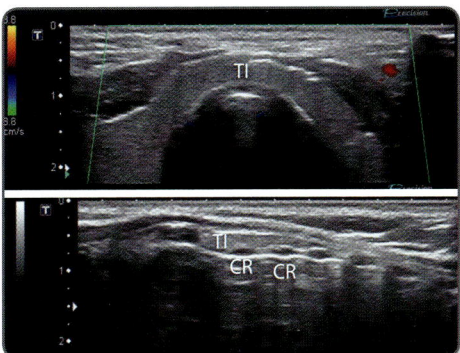

Figure 3.9 Ultrasound can be immediate and informative. Axial and sagittal imaging through the thyroid isthmus and trachea demonstrates the utility of ultrasound in visualizing the thyroid and superficial vasculature, particularly useful in procedure planning in the setting of coagulopathy. Red, superficial vessel; CR, tracheal cartilage ring; TI, thyroid isthmus.

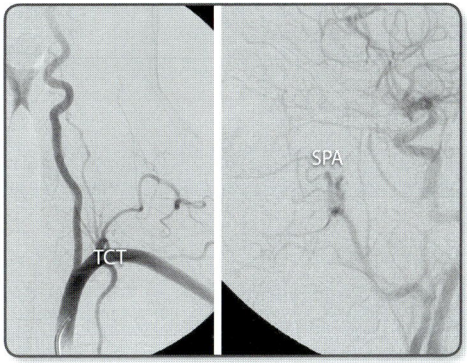

Figure 3.10 Angiography. On injection of the left subclavian artery and left common carotid artery, mapping the vasculature perfusing the airway can be easily done, but is often impractical and unnecessary with the availability of less invasive modalities. The greatest utility is in identifying and treating active bleeding in the acute or postoperative setting. SPA, sphenopalatine artery; TCT, thyrocervical trunk (most likely sharing an origin with the costocervical trunk).

Angiography and nuclear medicine

These modalities offer limited utility in airway assessment initially, but may occasionally be beneficial in complicated cases. Angiography involves the direct catheterization of blood vessels, usually via the femoral artery through the inguinal route, and injection of contrast under fluoroscopy (**Figure 3.10**). The risks of radiation exposure and drug reaction are managed by the operator. An angiographer may map patient vasculature or find the source for bleeding, particularly in the post-tracheostomy setting, with the added benefit of embolization if indicated. Both CT and MRI offer good, but imperfect, angiographic imaging, but without the ability to intervene in the acute setting. Changing trends in diagnostic radiology have begun to favor CT angiography as a screening modality, but catheter angiography remains the gold standard. Nuclear medicine offers little by way of demonstrating the central airway itself, but may aid in the search for occult infections, neoplasm characterization, and distribution (PET; positron emission tomography) or in locating cerebrospinal fluid leaks (**Figure 3.11**).

Special considerations

Medical imaging is now a more integral component of patient assessment and management, but it comes with a cost. As the integration of imaging becomes more prominent in medical management, the general population's radiation exposure has significantly increased, as demonstrated by its effects on cancer incidence. Furthermore, the risk

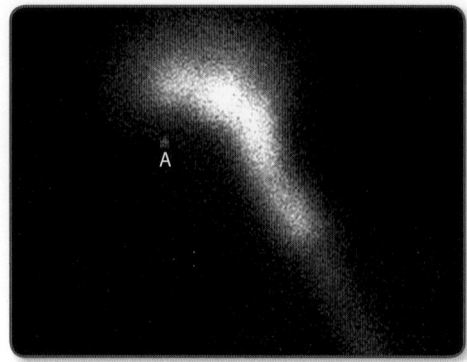

Figure 3.11 Nuclear medicine. Affectionately referred to as 'unclear medicine', it is traditionally reserved for diagnostic dilemmas. In this case of a simulated cerebrospinal fluid leak, abnormal activity (A) is seen in the anterior nasopharynx.

profile of imaging contrast agents is becoming clearer (ACR Manual on Contrast Media 2013). Finally, we are more frequently seeing our own limitations, for example in the over-diagnosis of incidental findings and in the degraded imaging of obese patients. It is in acknowledgment of these that we remember *primum non nocere* and recognize the guidance of our predecessor's dictum to 'treat the patient, not the images.'

If the outcome will not change your management, the test is unnecessary. Or put another way, any risk in the absence of a potential benefit is not worth taking.

Radiation safety and the pediatric population

Since the advent of radiology, medical radiation has surpassed background radiation, resulting in a small but real increase in the incidence of cancer. The study of these effects shows that dividing cells are more susceptible than nondividing cells, thus putting children at the greatest risks. In fact, the American College of Radiology, in conjunction with several other organizations, has created the Alliance for Radiation Safety in Pediatric Imaging, which promotes the 'Image Gently' campaign. Provided in their literature are several guidelines and imaging protocols optimized for children. In adults, imaging the airway increases exposure to the thyroid, breast tissue, and the eyes, all of which show increased sensitivity to radiation's effects. While no examination imparts enough radiation to significantly increase the risk of cancer, the cumulative dose over the life of the patient may be significant. Consequently, all clinicians should be aware of the potential consequences when imaging, not to prevent necessary imaging, but to limit unnecessary exposure to radiation.

Contrast media risks and benefits

Radiologists employ a myriad of agents to provide improved visualiz-ation of anatomy and pathology. When imaging the airway, possible agents include barium sulfate, iodinated oral suspension, intravenous iodinated agents, and chelated gadolinium agents. The oral agent gold standard is barium sulfate, but there is a relative contraindication in the setting of suspected perforation necessitating the iodinated alternative. If no perforation is detected with oral iodinated contrast medium, the examination may be completed with barium sulfate, in order to attain maximum sensitivity. Intravenous contrast risks are often more significant. Though rare, anaphylactic reactions to intravenous contrast do occur. While occasionally suspected in atopic patients, the best predictor is a history of prior reaction. Once an allergy is known, premedication for 12–24 hours allows for the safest examination. According to the American College of Radiology, a frequently used premedication routine includes 50 mg of oral prednisone at 13, 7, and 1 hour prior to the examination in addition to 50 mg of oral diphenhydramine 1 hour prior to the examination. In the emergent setting, 40 mg of methylprednisolone sodium succinate intravenously every 4 hours prior to the examination (for as long as a patient can wait up to the 13 hour regimen) provides some protection, but premedicating <6 hours prior to the administration of contrast has not shown efficacy. Of note, there is no known cross-reaction between iodine-based (CT) and gadolinium (MR) contrast agents, a distinction often misunderstood by patients. Iodinated contrast agents also increase the risk of renal injury if the patient already has renal insufficiency and lactic acidosis if the patient is on metformin. In contrast, gadolinium products have been associated with nephrogenic systemic fibrosis in renally impaired patients – a slowly progressive, and sometimes fatal, consequence.

Imaging limitations and consequences

With the continued integration of medical imaging into medical management, it is common to find referring physicians disappointed by an inadequate or overanalyzed image interpretation on the part of the radiologist. The etiology for any dissonance between the patient's presentation and the image results may result from a misunderstanding of the examination's indication, problems with patient cooperation, body habitus, and extraneous findings. Only through continuous communication can the examination and report be tailored in a way to maximize the benefit to the patients and their subsequent management. This communication is something that can be developed over time, and with multidisciplinary co-operation.

Now that digital radiography is replacing film, the two most common reasons for poor quality examinations are patient motion and body habitus. Patient motion can be minimized, if necessary, by medicating the patient, but in most cases, modern multidetector CT scanners can acquire adequate images in less than a minute, making this less of a problem than it was in the past. Multiple repeated attempts should be avoided to minimize patient radiation dose. MRI, on the other hand, is incredibly susceptible to motion. If a patient is uncooperative, the examination will be of limited use. Obesity—a growing epidemic—

impairs all modalities in a similar manner without good alternatives. Here as much as anywhere, patient presentation often trumps any imaging findings.

VOMIT is an acronym and euphemism adapted by many medical trainees defined as 'victims of medical imaging technology', referring to the limitless work-ups for incidental pulmonary and thyroid nodules discovered peripherally on patient examinations. CT and MRI find countless asymptomatic lesions without adequate criteria for differentiating benign from malignancy pathology, necessitating further workup. This workup may save a life or result in a series of adverse complications but benign lesions are typically more common. While the optimal approach is still controversial, cross-sectional imaging may open Pandora's box, generating excess anxiety in an already stressful situation.

References

ACR Committee on Drugs and Contrast Media. ACR Manual on Contrast Media, Version 9. ACR 2013; 8-9. http://www.acr.org/~/media/ACR/Documents/PDF/QualitySafety/Resources/Contrast%20Manual/2013_Contrast_Media.pdf

4 Anesthesia and management of the difficult airway

Howard R Bromley, Kerry C Snyder, Adryan Emion

Introduction

The failure to properly manage the serious challenge of the difficult airway can result in a chaotic situation unrivaled by few other clinical events.

The difficult airway can be defined several ways, with definitions including the level of experience of the medical personnel, repeated attempts at intubation, and whether a bougie or other intubation aid was used. Perhaps one of the most widely used classifications is by Cormack and Lehane (Cormack & Lehane 1984), which describes the best view of the larynx seen at laryngoscopy when there is visibility (**Figure 4.1**). Unfortunately, Cormack and Lehane's classification is of no use in situations where the larynx cannot be visualized, and it is not useful to predict a difficult intubation. It is used to record the visibility of the patient's airway for future reference.

Simply put, the difficult airway is defined as a clinical situation in which a caregiver experiences difficulty with mask ventilation, difficulty with tracheal intubation, or both (Caplan et al. 1993).

The overall incidence of encountering a difficult airway is estimated to be <10% of all cases of airway management (Crosby et al. 1998). However, it is apparent that the lack of planning for the possibility of

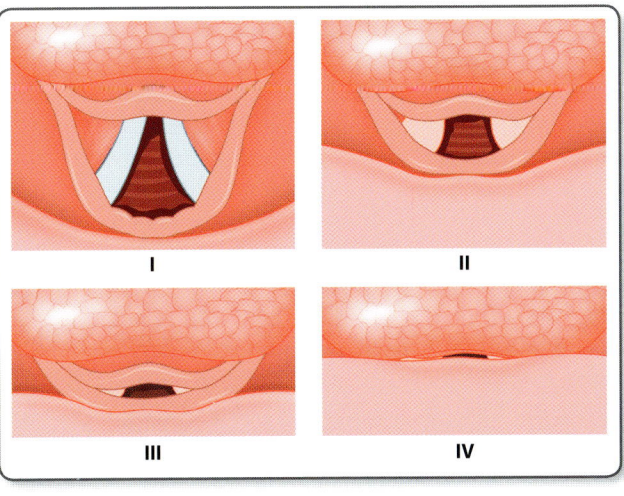

Figure 4.1 Cormack and Lehane's classification of laryngoscopy views. Class I: the vocal cords are visible; class II: the vocals cords are only partly visible; class III: only the epiglottis is seen; class IV: the epiglottis cannot be seen.

entering a difficult airway scenario is most often the cause of poor clinical outcomes (Roberts 1995). Unfortunately, there exists no single ideal or precise method of evaluating the airway prior to intubation.

The consequences of failure to intubate or secure an airway have been associated with serious complications such as hypoxemia, hypercapnia, resultant metabolic alterations, neurological sequelae including anoxia, and death.

Airway assessment

Any abnormalities of the bony structures of the jaw and/or face, and the soft tissues of the upper airway, can result in a difficult airway scenario. If you can predict a difficult airway, then you can properly prepare yourself for what may occur.

A thorough history and examination is paramount in discovering a difficult airway. Some obvious clinical situations that are likely to present as a difficult intubation include:

- Pregnant women and morbidly obese people (due to redundant tissue)
- Facial and/or maxillary/mandibular trauma
- Small mandibles, as there is decreased space for the tongue
- Intraoral pathology such as infections or tumors
- Inability to open the mouth
- Small mouth
- Poor teeth

Craniocervical movement

Patients who suffer from rheumatoid disease of the neck or degenerative spinal diseases such as ankylosing spondylitis will often have markedly reduced neck mobility. The inability of patients to fully extend their neck decreases their capability to obtain the classic 'sniffing the morning air' position and thus results in misalignment of the laryngeal and pharyngeal axes (**Figure 4.2**).

When properly positioned, all axes are aligned (**Figure 4.3**). To minimize excessive neck movement during intubation attempts, ask someone to hold the patient's head steady and provide inline stabilization while also delivering an upward bilateral jaw thrust.

A patient's history of prior successful or unsuccessful intubations is a significant predictor, but age may change this. There a number of specific clinical assessments that have been developed to try to identify patients who may prove to be difficult to intubate.

Mallampati suggested a simple screening test that is widely used today in a modified form (Samsoon & Young 1987). The patient sits or stands in front of the examiner and opens his or her mouth as widely as possible. The patient's airway is assigned a grade according to the best view obtained (see Figure 2.10). This test should not be performed with the patient supine, as gravity will force the tongue posteriorly, resulting in an inaccurate score.

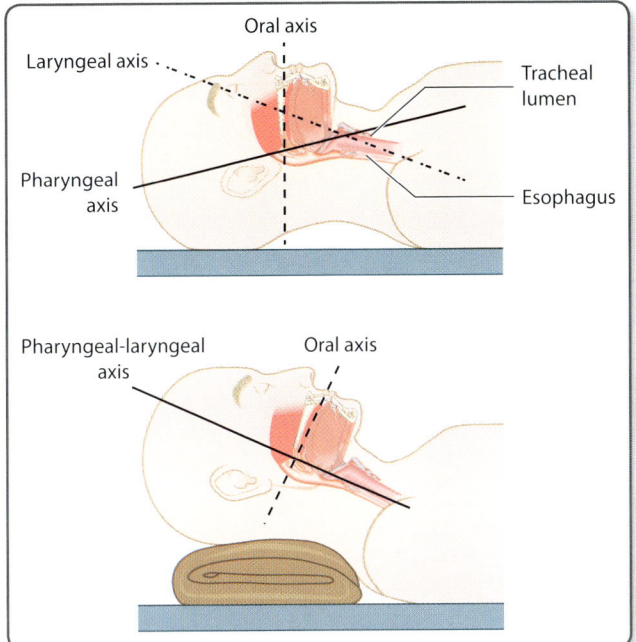

Oral axis

Laryngeal axis

Tracheal lumen

Pharyngeal axis

Esophagus

Pharyngeal-laryngeal axis

Oral axis

Figure 4.2 Alignment of airway axes. (a) Patient supine; all axes unaligned. (b) Neck forward, partially extended; pharyngeal and laryngeal axes aligned.

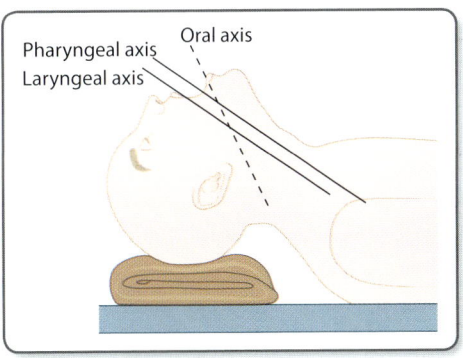

Oral axis

Pharyngeal axis
Laryngeal axis

Figure 4.3 Proper alignment of airway axes to view vocal cords.

The Mallampati test is scored as follows:
1. Faucial pillars, soft palate, and uvula easily visualized
2. Faucial pillars and soft palate visualized, but the uvula is masked by the base of the tongue
3. Only the soft palate is visualized
4. Soft palate is not seen and is obscured by the tongue

Clinically, grade 1 usually means that the patient will be easy to intubate, and grade 3 or 4 suggests a high chance that the patient will prove difficult to intubate. The results of the Mallampati test are influenced by patient position, mouth opening, tongue size and mobility, and movement at the craniocervical junction.

Thyromental distance

This is the measurement taken from the thyroid cartilage notch to the tip of the mandible with the head slightly extended. If the distance is >6.5 cm, conventional intubation is usually possible. If it is <6 cm, intubation may be difficult (Patil et al. 1983). Freck showed that by combining the modified Mallampati score and thyromental distance, patients who fulfilled the criteria of a grade 3 or 4 on the Mallampati score and who also had a thyromental distance of <7 cm were likely to present difficulty with intubation (Freck 1991).

Prognostication

Protrusion of the mandible (prognostication) is an indication of the mobility of the mandible. If the patient is able to protrude the lower teeth beyond the upper incisors and bite the upper lip, intubation is predictably easy (Calder et al. 1995). If the patient cannot prognosticate, intubation is likely to be difficult.

Mandibular space

In the supine position during laryngoscopy, the patient's tongue is lifted up into the mandibular space. If the patient's tongue is too big, or the mandibular space is too small, then either issue or both will lead to the tongue intruding into the oral space and likely obscuring the laryngoscopist's view.

A combination of tests is better than using only one. The modified Mallampati score, thyromental distance, ability to protrude the mandible, mandibular space, and craniocervical movement are the most reliable indicators.

ASA difficult airway algorithm

The American Society of Anesthesiologists (ASA) has developed an algorithm (**Figure 4.4**) for handling difficult airways. It is composed of two basic limbs: one dealing with the recognized or anticipated difficult airway and the other addressing the unrecognized condition. Any practitioner who is routinely confronted with intubating a patient should be familiar with this algorithm.

Approach to management

Practitioners must become proficient with a variety of airway alternatives in a nonemergent environment conducive to learning and practicing their skills. Practitioners must be able to work within a respectful team dynamic, manage a critical situation, and make decisions while moving through a predetermined difficult airway plan. The ultimate management goal is to safely secure the airway while maintaining oxygenation. Plans must include alternatives for management of the predicted difficult airway as well as the 'can't intubate, can't ventilate' scenario. Kits that are portable, comprehensive, and well-maintained

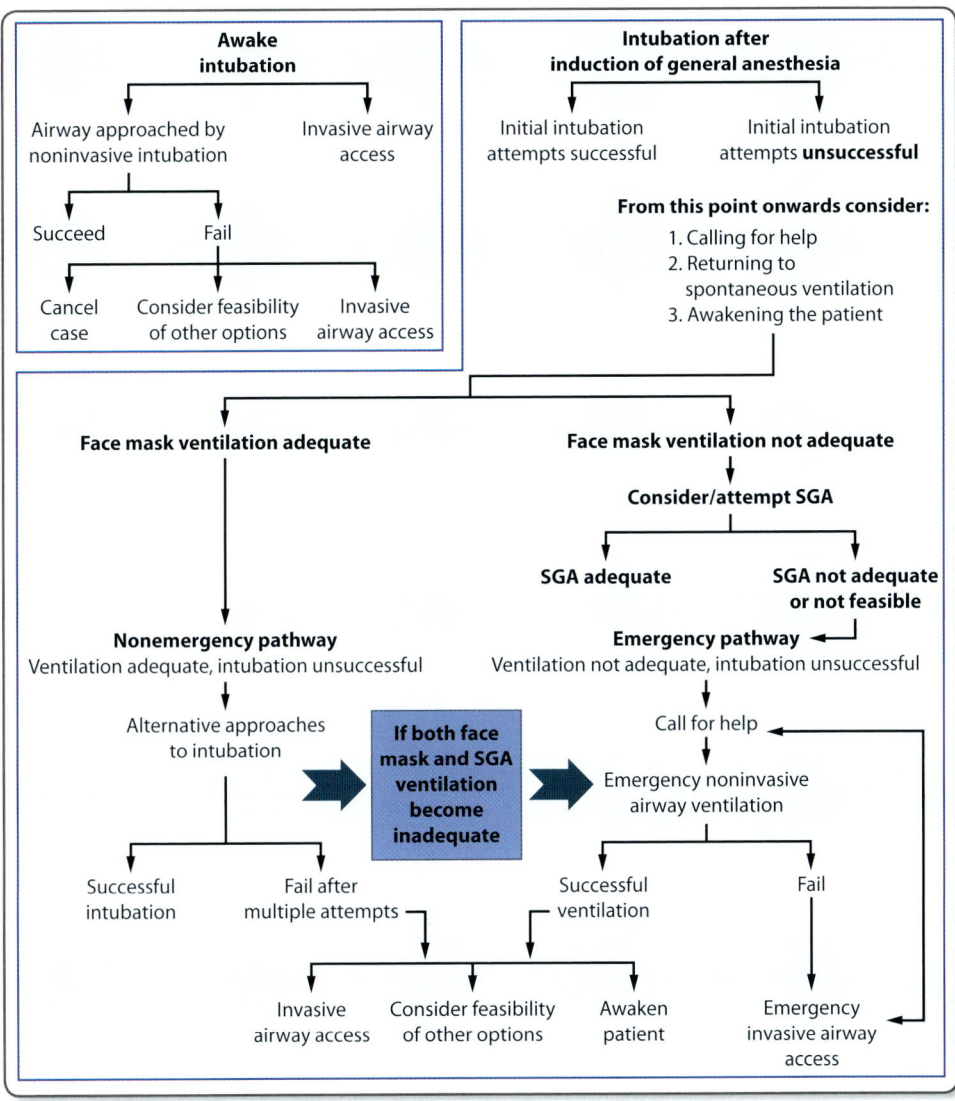

Figure 4.4 American Society of Anesthesiologists difficult airway algorithm. SGA, supraglottic airway (e.g. a laryngeal mask airway). With permission from: Apfelbaum JL, Hagberg CA, Caplan RA, et al. Practice Guidelines for Management of the Difficult Airway: An updated report by the American Society of Anesthesiologists Task Force on management of the difficult airway. Anesthesiology 2013; 118:251–270.

provide practitioners with multiple alternatives. These should include but not be limited to suction, oxygen delivery devices, bag-valve-mask ventilation devices, oral and nasal airways, multiple sized laryngoscopes, endotracheal tubes (ETT), airway exchange catheters, bougies, carbon dioxide detectors, a fiberoptic/video laryngoscope, rescue airways, and surgical airway supplies. Selection of a limited number of these airway devices allows practitioners to become proficient with their use and placement.

Since the assessment of the airway may be abbreviated due to circumstances, a prior intubation history can be valuable if attainable. If it is determined that an airway may be difficult to intubate, consideration should be given to performing an awake intubation if not contraindicated. If time allows, the patient should be prepared psychologically and pharmacologically for an awake intervention (Rumkumar 2011). Prior to induction and intubation, patients should be preoxygenated for 3 minutes if possible to increase the blood oxygen saturation and delay significant drops in saturation during intubation (Mort 2004). Alternately, preoxygenation with four maximal breaths in 30 seconds will provide similar starting oxygen saturation levels, but desaturation may occur more quickly (Apfelbaum et al. 2013).

Medical contraindications, allergies, volume status, comorbidities, and overall condition should contribute to the selection of induction agents. Induction agents should be sufficient to provide optimal intubating conditions, because the incidence of airway-related complications increases with subsequent attempts (Mort 2004). The decision to move forward to alternative interventions should be made early when conventional efforts at laryngoscopy fail.

Patients should be monitored during intubation efforts including pulse oximetry. Oxygen saturation should be monitored closely with predetermined cutoff points to stop and ventilate/oxygenate. When oxygen saturation drops to 90%, the descent after that point is often rapid and recovery may be delayed, even with positive pressure ventilation (Mort 2004).

When a particularly ominous airway situation presents itself, it is prudent to consider a surgical airway intervention. Decisions are based on patient condition, airway assessment, and ease of surgical airway placement. The option may be to attempt an awake or asleep 'look' or to proceed directly with a surgical airway.

Nonsurgical cricothyrotomy may be attempted by needle cricothyrotomy utilizing an intravenous catheter, but this technique has a high failure and complication rate (Mort 2007). The percutaneous placement of a wide-bore cannula through the cricothyroid membrane utilizing the Seldinger technique may offer a method with a higher comfort level for nonsurgical providers (Mort 2007).

Anesthetizing the airway and techniques

It is imperative that the patient is cooperative and ventilation is maintained throughout the process to prevent a difficult situation from evolving into a dangerous one. The airway should ideally be free of any fluids including blood and saliva that would impair visualization of the airway, and adequately topically anesthetized in awake patients. There are many different methods of topically anesthetizing the airway, and techniques will vary among individuals according to experience and personal beliefs about efficacy.

Agents and techniques

Glycopyrolate (0.2–0.4 mg intravenous) is an antimuscarinic agent with potent antisialagogue activity, allowing the local anesthetic agents more contact time with the oral mucosa. Glycopyrrolate should be administered 20–30 minutes before topical anesthetics so that salivary function is adequately impaired (Pai et al. 2001). Once the airway is topically anesthetized, the practitioner should ideally perform the airway management before the effects of the local anesthetics diminish.

Lidocaine 5% ointment may be applied to the distal third of a tongue blade and placed as far back in the patient's mouth as tolerable so that the lidocaine contacts the posterior tongue. The patient then clenches his teeth on the tongue blade to hold it in place. Through a combination of melting, gravity, and swallowing, the ointment will be distributed in the posterior pharynx in approximately 10 minutes. Lidocaine 2% liquid or viscous may be swished and gargled by the patient and then swallowed.

Nebulized lidocaine may be used to prepare the airway for manipulation with 5 mL of 4% lidocaine via facemask or mouthpiece. Benzocaine spray may also be used in small amounts to anesthetize the oral mucosa, but it must be used sparingly as its use is limited due to possible methemoglobinemia (Taleb et al. 2013). If nebulization is not performed, it may be desirable to perform a transtracheal block using 3–4 mL of 4% lidocaine administered through the cricothyroid membrane to help prevent coughing and vocal cord spasm during the intubation of awake patients.

Both the nasopharynx and the oropharynx should be topically prepared for a nasotracheal approach. Bleeding is a common concern: to reduce the risk of bleeding, a topical atomized vasoconstrictor such as oxymetazolone should be administered to both nares, so that the contralateral side may be utilized if necessary. Prewarming of the ETT may reduce bleeding and damage in the nasopharynx (Yong et al. 2000). Lidocaine gel 2% or ointment 5% can be applied to the nasal mucosa several minutes prior to intubation to increase the patient's comfort.

The 'awake look'

If the practitioner suspects that there may be a chance that a traditional laryngoscopy might be successful, a technique called the 'awake look' may be utilized for assessment of the airway. Since direct laryngoscopy may activate the gag reflex and cause a hemodynamic response, the patient's oropharynx should be topically anesthetized. The 'awake look' consists of a gentle, brief laryngoscopy to assess which airway structures may be viewed. The BURP (backward upward rightward pressure) technique (Knill 1993) may be used to move the thyroid cartilage posterior, cephalad, and toward the patient's right side. This technique may be useful to reposition the anterior glottis into view during awake or asleep laryngoscopy.

Blind nasal intubation

Useful in awake or sedated spontaneously breathing patients, blind nasal intubations don't require additional equipment other than an ETT. The ETT should be introduced into a nare and slowly advanced until fogging is seen and breath sounds are heard in the tube, indicating that the tip is very near the glottic opening. Timed with inspiration, the ETT is quickly advanced. If in the trachea, this will almost always result in significant coughing and obvious air movement through the ETT. If there is inadvertent esophageal placement indicated by a lack of breath impulses, the tube may be withdrawn until the breath sounds are just reacquired, and the method repeated.

Video laryngoscope and fiberoptic bronchoscope

The video laryngoscope has evolved into an extremely valuable tool in the management of difficult airways. With the camera positioned at the distal tip of the blade, the anterior glottis is easily visualized without the need to align the laryngeal and oral axes. Flexible fiberoptic bronchoscopes (FOB) may be used for both oral and nasal approaches to the difficult airway. A standard ETT may be preloaded onto the FOB. Upon advancement of the FOB past the vocal cords into the trachea, the ETT is guided captively into the trachea over the scope. A medium-sized bronchoscope has the advantage of a larger suction channel to clear secretions from the oropharynx.

In situations where the FOB is of limited use related to unidentifiable or swollen airway anatomy, a combination technique using video laryngoscopy and fiber optic intubation may prove useful. One practitioner places the video laryngoscope in the mouth to obtain a view of the glottis, while a second practitioner guides the FOB either orally or nasally into the view of the video monitor. The ETT is then advanced over the FOB into the trachea as viewed on the video laryngoscope monitor.

Rescue airways

Preparation for the 'can't intubate, can't ventilate' event must include the immediate availability of rescue airway devices. Features of these devices include placement without the use of laryngoscopy or visualization, a high success level in placement, and allowance for oxygenation and ventilation while the patient is allowed to wake up, or a more definitive airway plan is put in place. Commonly used rescue airways include a variety of supraglottic devices as well as variations on esophageal obturators (EOs).

The most commonly used supraglottic airway is the laryngeal mask airway (LMA), which appears as part of the ASA Difficult Airway Algorithm in the case of inability to intubate and inadequate face mask ventilation (Law et al. 2013). Variations include a variety of cuff configurations, disposable or reusable LMAs, gastric drainage ports, and those that allow endotracheal intubation while in situ. LMAs are often used by providers as an alternative to face mask ventilation during an anesthetic and as a rescue device when conventional intubation techniques fail. There is an associated learning curve to their successful placement (Zundert et al. 2012). The most common cause of placement failure of an LMA is a small oral aperture, short, thick neck, large tongue, blood/mucus in the mouth and retrognathy (Zundert et al. 2012). Since there is no occlusion of the esophagus with the LMA, there is no protection against aspiration of gastric contents and it should be replaced when appropriate with a definitive airway for long-term ventilation.

Intubation through the LMA is possible with the Fastrach LMA or by the use of an Aintree Intubation Catheter (AIC) through which a fiberoptic intubating scope is placed. Proper placement of the device will ideally allow the Fastrach ETT to be passed through the lumen of the LMA into the trachea. After intubation, the Fastrach may be left in place temporarily or removed by using the pusher rod supplied with the kit.

EOs allow prehospital providers who are untrained in endotracheal intubation to rapidly secure the airway. The King Laryngeal Tube (King LT) is a single lumen device with a closed end that is placed into the oropharynx and blindly passed into the esophagus. Occlusive balloons are inflated in the esophagus and pharynx, and the patient is ventilated through supraglottic lumens. The possibility exists to place the lumen in the trachea that would prevent ventilation of the patient. If this occurs, the tube should be removed and replaced with manual anterior displacement of the trachea.

The Combitube is also inserted blindly. It has a dual cuff, dual tube design that allows for placement in either the esophagus or the trachea. The assumption is also that the tube will seat in the esophagus, but offers an alternative if tracheal placement occurs in that it does not occlude the trachea.

Any EO should not be placed in an alert patient or one with an intact gag reflex, and cannot be placed in patients with clenched teeth. They are contraindicated in patients with upper airway obstruction, known esophageal disease, or suspected tracheal injury (Zundert et al. 2012). EOs must be removed prior to endotracheal intubation in most cases. Possible complications of EO use include aspiration, soft tissue damage, tracheal or esophageal injury, and tongue swelling during prolonged use (Zundert et al. 2012).

Extubation

Knowing when to extubate is important and best done when the patient is awake and responsive. Various maneuvers can be utilized to validate extubation. Adequate spontaneous respiratory function with a vital capacity of >15 mL/kg and a negative inspiratory force of >20 Torr is recommended.

Airway edema may be assessed both audibly and visually prior to extubation. If air is heard escaping during positive pressure ventilation after the cuff is deflated (called the cuff leak test), then the patient is unlikely to have significant airway edema. If no escaping air is heard, extubation is not recommended.

For visual assessment of airway edema, the FOB can be placed in a nare and advanced until the ETT cuff is seen. Performing the cuff leak test then provides both an audible and a visual affirmation of an air leak. If significant tracheal edema is visualized, extubation should not proceed.

In the event that both of the above tests validate an acceptable air leak and minimal edema, but there is still a suspicion of airway problems, a bougie or AIC may be placed through the ETT prior to extubation. Lidocaine, 2% or 4%, 10 mL, should be administered down the ETT. The ETT may then be carefully removed, leaving the bougie or AIC in place in the event of the need for emergent reintubation. If the patient is breathing spontaneously without any evidence of upper airway edema after 30 minutes, the bougie or AIC may be removed.

Documentation

When a patient has had a difficult airway event, it is prudent to assume that future intubations will also be difficult, unless a significant change in the patient's status has occurred (e.g. weight, airway swelling, or cervical immobilization). Complete and thorough documentation including the number of attempts at intubation, ease of ventilation, other interventions, devices used, and intubation views throughout the event is the key to the prevention of future similar situations. Communication may be accomplished by a hospital-wide system of 'Difficult Airway' wristbands.

After a difficult airway event, a letter given to the patient regarding his or her airway history will provide other practitioners with the details of the event. The patients should be instructed to keep the letter with them and produce it on the occasion of future hospitalizations or surgeries.

Conclusion

While there is no single ideal or precise method of evaluating the airway prior to intubation, the ability to appreciate the issues of management of the airway will help medical personnel properly anticipate and plan for potential problems. Such prior and proper planning may help place providers in a position of a successfully secured airway, rather than that of a morbid outcome. Even in the most mundane clinical airway situations, backup plans, including videoscopy, FOB, and establishing an emergent surgical airway must always be considered.

Most patients without any difficult intubation indicators will prove easy to intubate, although occasional difficulties may still be encountered. The majority of difficult airways can be predicted by clinical assessment. However, none of these tests are 100% accurate and may erroneously predict a difficult intubation in some patients to whom intubation will subsequently prove to be uncomplicated. In the extreme case of the patient who could not be easily intubated or ventilated, the price of premature extubation may be serious and life threatening. Extra precautions should be taken prior to extubation.

Lastly, when a difficult intubation has been encountered, thorough documentation and proper communication may preclude a future repeat of the event.

References

Apfelbaum JL, Hagberg CA, Caplan RA, et al; American Society of Anesthesiologists Task Force on Management of the Difficult Airway. Practice guidelines for management of the difficult airway: an updated report by the American Society of Anesthesiologists Task Force on Management of the Difficult Airway. Anesthesiology 2013; 118:251–270.

Calder I, Calder J, Crockard HA. Difficult direct laryngoscopy in patients with cervical spine disease. Anaesthesia 1995; 50:756–763.

Caplan RA, Benumof JL, Berry FA, et al. Practice guidelines for management of the difficult airway. Anesthesiology 1993; 78:597–602.

Cormack RS, Lehane J. Difficult intubation in obstetrics. Anaesthesia 1984; 39:1105–1111.

Crosby ET, Cooper RM, Douglas MI, et al. The unanticipated difficult airway with recommendations for management. Can J Anaesth 1998; 45:757–776.

Freck CM. Predicting difficult intubation. Anaesthesia 1991; 46:1005–1008.

Knill RL. Difficult laryngoscopy made easy with a 'BURP.' Can J Anaesth 1993; 40:798–799.

Law JA, Broemling N, Cooper RM, et al. The difficult airway with recommendations for management – part 1– difficult tracheal intubation encountered in an unconscious/induced patient. Can J Anaesth 2013; 60:1089–1118.

Mort TC. Complications of emergency tracheal intubation: immediate airway-related consequences: Part II. J Intensive Care Med 2007; 22:208–215.

Mort TC. Emergency tracheal intubation: complications associated with repeated laryngoscopic attempts. Anesth Analg 2004; 99:607–613.

Pai S, Ghezzi EM, Ship JA. Development of a Visual Analogue Scale questionnaire for subjective assessment of salivary dysfunction. Oral Surg Oral Med Oral Pathol Oral Radiol Endod 2001; 91:311–316.

Patil VU, Stehling LC, Zaunder HL. Fiberoptic endoscopy in anesthesia. Chicago: Year Book Medical Publishers, 1983.

Roberts JT. Fundamentals of tracheal intubation. New York: Grune and Stratton, Inc., 1995:105–116.

Rumkumar V. Preparation of the patient and the airway for awake intubation. Indian J Anaesth 2011; 55:442–447.

Samsoon GLT, Young JRB. Difficult tracheal intubation: a retrospective study. Anaesthesia 1987; 42:487–490.

Taleb M, Ashraf Z, Valavoor S, et al. Evaluation and management of acquired methemoglobinemia associated with topical benzocaine use. Am J Cardiovasc Drugs 2013; 13:325–330.

Yong CK, Seung HL, Gyu JN, et al. Thermosoftening treatment of the nasotracheal tube before intubation can reduce epistaxis and nasal damage. Anesth Analg 2000; 91:698–701.

Zundert TV, Brimacombe JR, Ferson DZ, et al. Archie Brain: celebrating 30 years of development in laryngeal mask airways. Anaesthesia 2012; 67:1375–1385.

Indications and techniques for airway intervention and management

Francisco Vieira, Joshua W Wood

Introduction

Tracheotomy is one of the oldest and most-performed surgeries for critically ill patients. By performing a tracheotomy at an earlier stage in critical care patients who require prolonged mechanical ventilation, the duration of assisted ventilation and length of intensive care unit stay may be shortened (McWhorter 2003, Griffiths et al. 2005). The optimal timing for the tracheotomy to prevent complications remains controversial (De Leyn et al. 2007). However, in patients with impending airway obstruction and in patients who are anticipated to require endotracheal intubation of >10–14 days' duration, a tracheotomy is indicated (Goldenberg & Bhatti 2005).

Current indications for tracheotomy include (De Leyn et al. 2007):

- Acute upper airway obstruction
- Prolonged ventilatory support
- Bronchiopulmonary toilette
- Inability to intubate (after failure of endoscopic-assisted intubation)
- Adjunct to management of major chest or head and neck surgery in which long-term ventilation support is predicted

Multiple factors are involved in the process of decision making for undergoing a tracheotomy. Important considerations include whether it is an elective or emergent airway situation or whether the procedure should be performed under general anesthesia. In certain situations, inducing general anesthesia may cause a stable airway to become an unstable airway, thus precipitating an emergent situation. The patient's body habitus is also an important factor, and tracheostomy in the obese population is especially challenging. The surgeon must decide whether the patient would benefit from a temporary or a permanent tracheotomy. A large number of complications can be prevented by identifying those factors that may predispose to complicated airways. It is also imperative to identify previously compensating comorbidities and to use meticulous surgical technique.

The technique described below has been used successfully as elective procedure in critically ill patients (including obese patients) who require long-term intubation. It aggregates useful technical pearls that can be applied to the general patient population, and describes in detail 10 simple and effective steps to follow. It serves as a guideline for the trainee surgeon or resident to a rational, uncomplicated, and safe procedure in a controlled environment.

Instruments tray

- Backhaus towel clips, 7.6 cm ($\times$ 6)
- #15 blade with knife handle ($\times$ 2)
- Allis tissue holding forceps, 15.2 cm ($\times$ 2)
- Senn double-ended retractors, 16.0 cm ($\times$ 2)
- DeBakey forceps, 15.2 cm ($\times$ 2)
- Metzenbaum dissecting scissors, curved, 13.3 cm
- US retractors, 20.3 cm ($\times$ 2)
- Mosquito forceps, curved, 12.7 cm ($\times$ 3)
- Kelly forceps, curved, 13.9 cm ($\times$ 3)
- Kocher curved clamp, 13.9 cm ($\times$ 3)
- Peanut round sponge dissector, 3/8"´ 1/4" on C-5 holder ($\times$ 15)
- News tracheotomy hooks, 15.0 cm
- Mayo-Hegar needle holder, 15.2 cm
- 2/0 Ethicon Mersilk silk suture in 19 mm 3/8 curved, PS-2 reverse cutting needle
- Frazier suction tube 2.7 mm, 17 cm
- Mayo dissecting scissors, straight, 13.9 cm
- Mayo dissecting scissors, curved, 13.9 cm
- Yankauer suction tube (disposable)
- CSF $\times$ CFN cannula #6 or #7
- 2/0 nylon black monofil in 26 mm 3/8 curved, PS-2 reverse cutting needle ($\times$ 2)
- Transparent film dressing 10 $\times$ 12 cm (Tegaderm)

Pertinent anatomy

Structural anatomy from the skin surface to the trachea:
1. Skin, platysma muscle, and superficial cervical fascia
2. Bilateral branches of anterior jugular vein
3. Superficial layer of deep cervical fascia (or investing fascia)
4. Median raphe of sternohyoid and sternothyroid muscles
5. Pretracheal adipose tissue, inferior thyroid veins, and possible thyroid ima artery
6. Thyroid isthmus overlapping the level of second and/or third tracheal ring
7. Pretracheal fascia
8. Bilateral tracheo-esophageal groove and the recurrent laryngeal nerve
9. Innominate artery passes between trachea and manubrium upward and lateral to the upper margin of the right sternoclavicular joint

Tracheotomy technique for the adult patient

Step 1: Positioning and landmark identification

- The patient is placed in a supine position and the neck is prepared and draped using the usual sterile technique. The neck is hyperextended unless there are contraindications such as rheumatoid arthritis or the suspicion of cervical spine injury (Malata et al. 1996)
- The identification of landmarks is paramount and can be done with a marker pen (**Figure 5.1**)
    - An inferior midline sternal notch (or furcula of manubrium) mark
    - A horizontal cricoid cartilage mark
    - A superior thyroid cartilage notch mark
    - A straight line from sternal notch to thyroid notch is a reference of midline
- A 2.0–3.5 cm straight line incision mark is drawn in the midline, centered between the sternal notch and cricoid cartilage according to the body habitus of the patient (Pracy & Watkinson 2005) (**Figure 5.2**)

> **Pearl:** The goal is to enter the trachea between the second and third tracheal rings. High incisions close to the cricoid cartilage may pose a potential risk for tracheal stenosis. Conversely, when the incision is made too low, the risk of brachiocephalic trunk injury or parietal pleura tear resulting in pneumothorax is increased (De Leyn et al. 2007).

Step 2: Skin incision

- Infiltration of local anesthesia (1% lidocaine) and 100,000 IU of epinephrine
- A scalpel incision of 2.0–4.0 cm according to the body habitus is placed vertically in the midline as previously marked

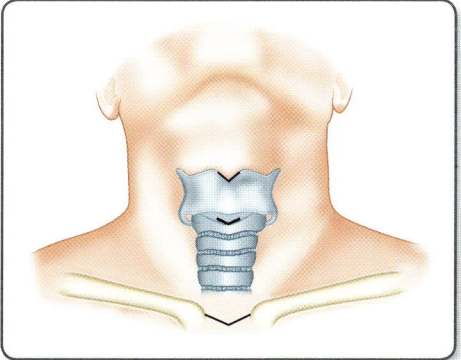

Figure 5.1 Tracheotomy surgical landmarks. Skin markings showing the thyroid and cricoid cartilages.

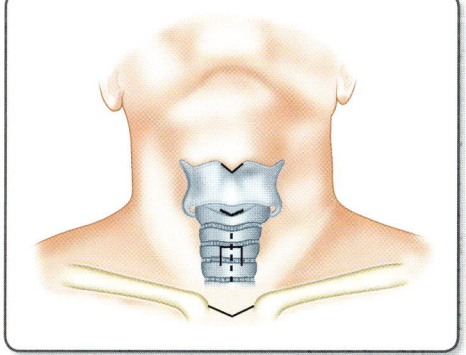

Figure 5.2 Tracheotomy surgical landmarks. Skin markings showing a vertical incision line.

- A midline incision should encompass the planes of the skin, subcutaneous tissue, platysma, and superficial cervical fascia

> **Pearl:** A horizontal incision may be used as well, depending on the surgeon's preference. In educational institutions, some surgeons recommend a vertical incision, which has fewer major vessels in the line of the incision and allows easier retraction of the strap muscles out of the line of the incision (Scurry & McGinn 2007). Many authors advocate that the direction of the incision does not affect the outcome, either functionally or cosmetically, and that the tracheostomy cannula size, duration, and local care are all more responsible for the resulting scar (Malata et al. 1996).

Step 3: Lipectomy

- The incision through the subcutaneous adipose tissue should meet the plane of the superficial layer of deep cervical fascia (or investing fascia)
- The obese patient will present a thick layer of adipose tissue at this level. With the help of a Senn retractor to give sufficient exposure, and the use of Allis forceps, a limited lipectomy can be achieved by the use of Bovie electrocautery (**Figure 5.3**)
- Once the adipose tissue is excised, the strap muscles are clearly visualized

> **Pearl:** The advantages of lipectomy in obese patients are (Gross et al. 2002):
> - Decreasing the risk of development of a false tract
> - Expediting cannula reinsertion in case of accidental decannulation
> - Allowing the placement of a standard tracheotomy tube
>   The disadvantage of lipectomy is:
> - Higher periostomal infection, since a larger dead space is created around the stoma

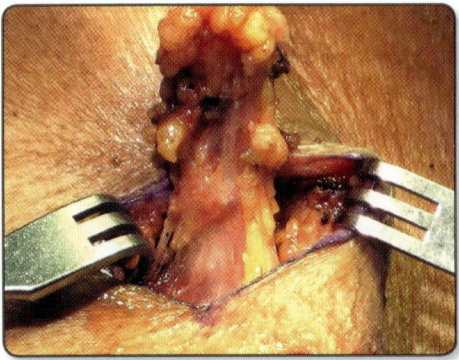 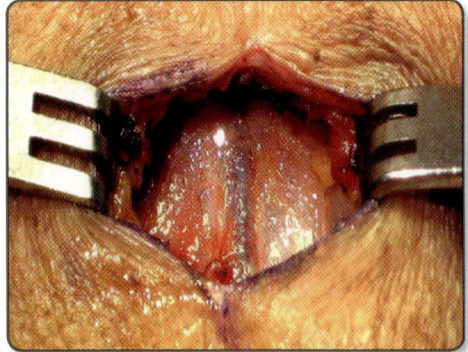

Figure 5.3 Lipectomy. Surgical picture showing the removal of fat tissue anterior to the trachea in an obese patient.

Figure 5.4 Strap muscle exposure. Surgical view of the sternohyoid and sternothyroid muscles, and the median raphe.

Step 4: Strap muscle dissection and retraction

- Once the sternohyoid muscle is visualized, the midline raphe is identified (**Figure 5.4**)
- With a help of DeBakey forceps, the raphe of the strap muscle is incised with electrocautery
- US Army-Navy retractors are repositioned to retract the strap muscles laterally

Step 5: Thyroid isthmus management and tracheal exposure

- At this point, the isthmus of the thyroid gland is exposed and a segment of trachea may be identified in various degrees above or below the second or third tracheal ring. The isthmus is divided in the midline and retracted laterally to minimize the risk of tube dislodgment during swallowing and pressure on the anterior tracheal wall (Calhoun et al. 1994)
- To split the isthmus, a right angle forceps is inserted underneath the isthmus plane to undermine and retract it superiorly (Calhoun et al. 1994) (**Figure 5.5**)
- Electrocautery in zigzag movements will help to split the isthmus safely in the midline above the pretracheal fascia plan (Scurry & McGinn 2007)
- Once the isthmus is divided, a Kittner dissector can be used to push away any residual soft tissue and the pretracheal fascia, allowing exposure of the tracheal wall
- At this step, hemostasis should be reviewed meticulously

> **Pearl:** If the second or third tracheal ring is deep to the substernal level, a cricoid hook should be used to retract the trachea superiorly, facilitating the dissection of the overlying tissue.

Step 6: Outlining the flap and stay suture placement with closed trachea

- If an endotracheal tube is being used for patient ventilation:
  - The anesthesiologist removes any tapes or ties used to secure the endotracheal tube, deflates the cuff, and advances it

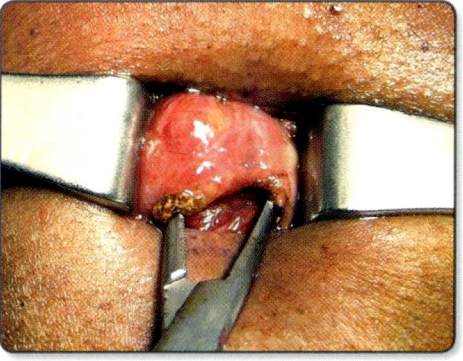

Figure 5.5 Thyroid isthmus. Surgical technique for exposing the thyroid isthmus with a right angle forceps.

distally toward the carina about 3.5 cm (1.5 inches) and then re-inflates the cuff

– Start decreasing FIO_2 to <30%

- A 2-0 silk stay suture is passed through the skin at the midline and the inferior aspect of the stoma and is then passed into the lumen of the trachea just below the second or third tracheal ring: it is then brought out above the tracheal ring to make a cartilaginous 'trap door flap' (Bjork flap) (Malata et al. 1996)
- Once the suture has been placed through the tracheal ring, it will follow a reverse pathway to the subcutaneous tissue and skin surface at the midline (**Figure 5.6**)

> **Pearl:** At this point, careful revision of hemostasis should be undertaken in in a meticulous manner. Since the trachea remains sealed and the FIO_2 is low, the use of Bovie cautery is safe throughout this step.

Step 7: Tracheal lumen exposure

- Once the surgical field is cleared of any bleeding, which mainly arises from the thyroid isthmus, electrocautery is used to delineate (over the pretracheal fascia) a midline inferior-based Bjork flap
- A scalpel blade is then used to complete the cartilage incision (**Figure 5.7**)
- In cases when the cartilage is abnormally thick or calcified, Mayo scissors can help to complete the incision and expose the tracheal lumen
- The low concentration of FIO_2 should be confirmed by the anesthesiologist
- The silk stay suture can be retracted to test the Bjork flap (**Figure 5.8**)

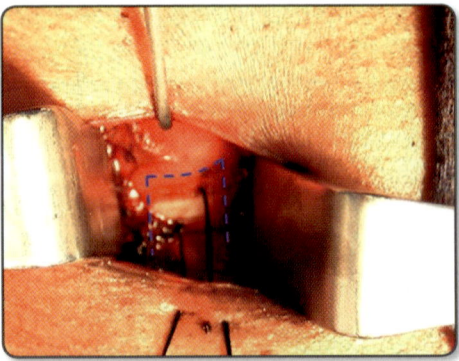

Figure 5.6 Placement of stay suture. Surgical view outlining the inferiorly based Bjork flap, as well as the proper placement of the stay suture.

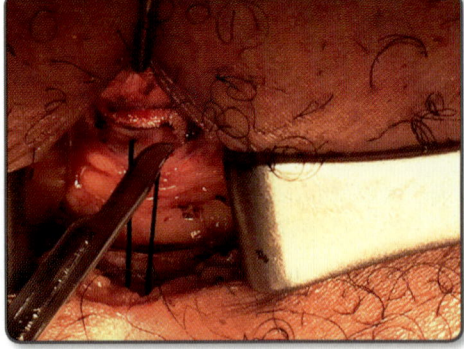

Figure 5.7 Tracheal lumen exposure. Surgical picture showing the exposure of the tracheal lumen with the use of a scalpel blade.

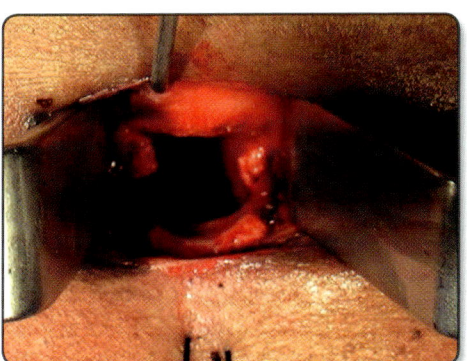

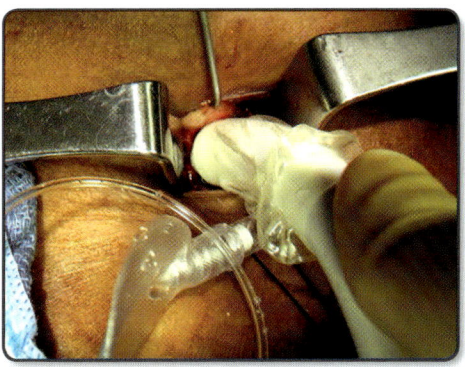

Figure 5.8 Inferiorly based Bjork flap. After the creation of the inferior-based Bjork flap, the previously placed stay suture is used to open the window into the tracheal lumen.

Figure 5.9 Insertion of tracheotomy cannula. Picture showing the easy insertion of the tracheotomy cannula after the creation of the Bjork flap.

> **Pearl:** Attention should be taken during this step to avoid puncturing or tearing the endotracheal tube cuff, which remains inflated during this step.

Step 8: Hemostasis control

- The anesthesiologist is asked to deflate the cuff and withdraw the tube to the level just above the stoma
- Once the field is inspected for bleeding, a suctioning tip can gently be introduced through the stoma site to collect any blood clots or secretions and evacuate any excess flammable O_2 remaining in the tracheal lumen
- Short bursts of electrocautery at a lower setting, or bipolar electrocautery, can be used to complete hemostasis in a safe way (Thompson et al. 1998)

> **Pearl:** In cases where the FiO_2 concentration cannot be lowered, a wet cloth should be kept by the scrub technician as a precautionary measure. In certain cases, silver nitrate sticks can be used judiciously to cauterize small vessels.

Step 9: Tracheal cannula insertion

- The tracheotomy cannula with its obturator is then gently inserted to fit the stoma without tightness. The cuff seal must be tested prior to insertion (**Figure 5.9**)
- The obturator is removed, and the inner cannula is inserted
- The cuff is then softly inflated by the surgeon or assistant, while the retractors remain in place

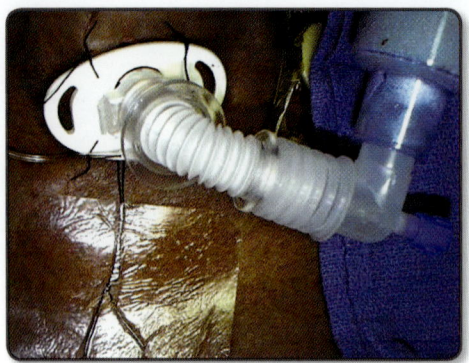

Figure 5.10 Connection of anesthesia circuit.

> **Pearl:** One should keep in mind that the adequate size of the cannula should be about two thirds, or no larger than three quarters, of the tracheal lumen diameter (Heffner et al. 1986). Different sizes should readily be available. For obese patients in particular, extra-long sizes, including proximal or distal extra length, may be required according to the patient's body habitus.

Step 10: Circuit reestablishment and securing the tube

- The anesthesia circuit is connected to the tracheostomy cannula, and the FiO_2 is raised. A normal tidal volume is re-established and confirmed by the anesthesiologist (**Figure 5.10**)
- The endotracheal tube and retractors are then completely removed
- Finally, a stay suture is placed securing the cannula flange to the superficial skin at four points using 2-0 nylon suture
- The silk suture from Bjork flap is tied about 0.5 cm from the skin, which allows for expansion of the skin due to edema. A tracheal tie is then placed and adjusted around the neck

> **Pearl:** A small Surgicel strip can be placed between the cannula and soft tissue. However, the skin incision should not be approximated. An open stoma allows loose space around the tube and minimizes the development of subcutaneous emphysema (Lai & Weinstein 2003). A Tegaderm dressing can be used to secure the silk suture to the chest skin for fast Bjork flap identification in case of reinsertion.

Pitfalls

Postoperative bleeding may be brisk from vascular origin, or it may be intermittent with small volume from the thyroid gland. The former requires control by digital pressure and prompt identification in the operating room, while the latter may be controlled at the bedside in most cases. Bleeding can be minimized by performing a Valsalva maneuver at the end of the procedure to identify any remaining bleeding vessels.

Chest radiographs should be obtained after emergent or difficult procedures, after placement of a low tracheotomy, in patients with emphysema, and in patients with progressing signs or symptoms of pneumothorax. However, they are not routinely necessary.

The development of a false tract is a life-threatening condition when not identified and can be prevented by the placement of four quadrant stay sutures securing the flange of the cannula to the superficial skin.

Subcutaneous emphysema can progress to mediastinal emphysema and can be prevented by not suturing the skin around the cannula.

Patients with shortness of breath in the immediate postoperative period should be investigated for a mucous plug. The inner cannula should be removed, and the patient should be suctioned with a flexible suction tip into the tracheostomy cannula. If the shortness of breath persists, dislodgment or a false tract should be considered. Removal of the cannula with prompt reinsertion of a new tracheotomy cannula should be attempted. Mucous plugs can be avoided by tracheal humidification.

If an urgent surgical airway is required, cricothyrotomy is well-established as the procedure of choice. Once stabilized, the cricothyrotomy should be replaced within 72 hours by a standard tracheotomy to avoid subglottic stenosis (Boon et al. 2004). If the patient has already had an endotracheal tube in place for >72 hours, then the cricothyrotomy should be replaced in 24–48 hours (Yuen et al. 2007).

Follow-up and recommendations

In an accidental postoperative decannulation, gentle traction of the silk stay suture will open the tracheal flap wide enough to reinsert the cannula and avoid the development of a false tract (Malata et al. 1996). After 5–7 days of the cannula being in place, the tracheostomy mucosa

Table 5.1 Tracheotomy complications		
Intraoperative	**Early postoperative**	**Late postoperative**
Bleeding (isthmus and vessels)	Tube obstruction (displacement/mucus plug)	Tracheal stenosis
Tube obstruction (malposition)	Accidental decannulation	Hemorrhage (innominate artery)
Fire ignition	False traject Bleeding (persistent oozing)	Peritracheal infection
Surgical emphysema	Surgical emphysema	Tube obstruction (displacement/mucus plug)
	Pneumothorax/pneumomediastinum	Accidental decannulation
		False traject Tracheoesophageal fistula
		Peritracheal granuloma

is mature enough to form a tract. The stay suture can be removed, and the tracheostomy cannula replaced (Scurry & McGinn 2007). Some authors recommend waiting a week for the creation of the stoma (De Leyn et al. 2007).

The tracheostomy tube cuff pressure should be in the range of 20-25 cmH$_2$O. Lower pressures can cause an air leak by longitudinal folding of the cuff and excessive mobilization against the tracheal mucosa. High cuff pressure causes capillary ischemia with tracheal mucosa damage, and may later result in tracheal stenosis.

Patient and caregiver education about tracheotomy maintenance and troubleshooting should be a part of the care for patients and should be addressed by the surgeon (Pracy & Watkinson 2005).

It is necessary to irrigate the tracheostomy cannula at least once a day with saline solution to avoid granulation tissue formation and potential infection. Tracheostomy tube assessment and local care with peristomal hygiene management at least twice a day are required.

There are a variety of complications that can arise following a tracheotomy. These are summarized in **Table 5.1**.

References

Boon JM, Abrahams PH, Meiring JH, et al. Cricothyroidotomy: a clinical anatomy review. Clin Anat 2004; 17:478–486.

Calhoun KH, Weiss RL, Scot B, et al. Management of the thyroid isthmus in tracheostomy: a prospective and retrospective study. Otolaryngol Head Neck Surg 1994; 111:450–452.

De Leyn P, Bedert L, Delcroix M, et al. Tracheotomy: clinical review and guidelines. Eur J Cardiothorac Surg 2007; 32:412–421.

Goldenberg D, Bhatti N. Management of the impaired airway in the adult. Cummings CW, Flint PW, Haughey BH, et al. (eds), Otolaryngology: head & neck surgery, 4th edn, Vol 3. Philadelphia: Mosby, 2005:2441–2453.

Griffiths J, Morgan L, Young J D. Systematic review and meta-analysis of studies of the timing of tracheostomy in adult patients undergoing artificial ventilation. BMJ 2005; 330:1243–1246.

Gross ND, Cohen JI, Andersen PE, et al. 'Defatting' tracheotomy in morbidly obese patients. Laryngoscope 2002; 112:1940–1944.

Heffner JE, Miller KS, Sahn S A, et al. Tracheostomy in the intensive care unit. Part 1: indications, technique, management. Chest 1986; 90:269–274.

Heffner JE, Miller SK, Sahn SA. Tracheostomy in the intensive care unit. Part 2: complications. Chest 1986; 90:430–436.

Lai SY, Weinstein GS. Tracheostomy demystifying an ancient technique. Operat Tech Otolaryngol Head Neck Surg 2003; 14:51–54.

Malata CM, Foo IT, Simpson KH, et al. An audit of Bjork flap tracheostomies in head and neck plastic surgery. Br J Oral Maxillofac Surg 1996; 34:42–46.

McWhorter AJ. Tracheotomy: timing and techniques. Curr Opin Otolaryngol Head Neck Surg 2003; 11:473–479.

Pracy JP, Watkinson JC. Surgical tracheostomy: how I do it. Ann R Coll Surg Engl 2005; 87: 285–287.

Scurry WC, McGinn JD. Operative tracheotomy. Operat Tech Otolaryngol Head Neck Surg 2007; 18:85–89.

Thompson JW, Colin W, Snowden T, et al. Fire in the operating room during tracheotomy. South Med J 1998; 91:243–247.

Yuen HW, Loy AH, Johari S. Urgent awake tracheotomy for impending airway obstruction. Otolaryngol Head Neck Surg 2007; 136:838–842.

6 Surgical management of the airway in the emergency department

R Mario Vera, Martin A Croce

Introduction

Evaluation of patients in the emergency department with potential airway compromise can be one of the most stressful and challenging clinical situations for the consultant surgeon. Initial evaluation of both the trauma patient and critically ill surgical patient must begin with an expedient but thorough evaluation of the airway. The decision to obtain surgical access to the airway must remain foremost in the surgeon's mind throughout the patient's stay in the emergency department.

Pre-emergency department management

Many critically ill patients arrive in the emergency department with airway access already obtained by prehospital providers. While each locality has its established set of protocols that dictate specific indications for the use of nasal, oral, supraglottic, or endotracheal airway devices, certain principles are common.

Indications for prehospital intervention are shown in **Box 6.1.** Prehospital providers must be skilled in the use of nasal and oral airways, supraglottic devices such as the laryngeal mask airway (LMA), and of course, the orally or nasally placed endotracheal tube (Berlac et al. 2008).

Necessary equipment for prehospital intubation includes appropriate intravenous sedatives and analgesics, oral and nasal airways of different sizes, endotracheal tubes of various sizes, laryngoscopes with properly functioning batteries, and various Macintosh and Miller blades.

Box 6.1 Indications for prehospital intubation
- Glasgow Coma Scale < 8
- Inability to protect airway
- Poor respiratory effort
- Cardiac or respiratory arrest

Management of the acute airway as dictated by Advanced Cardiac Life Support requires immediate evaluation and the readiness to act. Respiratory arrest should be addressed with the following:

- Providing supplemental oxygen
- Opening the airway
- Providing basic ventilation
- Ventilation via artificial airways
- The use of advanced airways

It is not uncommon for patients to present with impending airway compromise and thus to represent a challenging clinical scenario. While each clinical situation requires an individual and tailored response, it is prudent to act quickly when airway collapse is believed to be impending. In most situations, this means following the paradigm of early intubation when potential airway compromise is expected. Often, emergency providers will implement 'airway precautions,' a nebulous term that is wrought with potential for disaster. Given the grave consequences that can be associated with airway emergencies, it is the authors' practice to obtain a secure airway via endotracheal intubation early if potential airway compromise is even suspected.

Awake intubation versus the use of sedation

Patients with the high suspicion of a difficult airway present a unique clinical challenge. A difficult airway should be suspected in those with significant injury or distorted anatomy (**Box 6.2**). Patients who are obtunded, in cardiac or respiratory arrest, or in extremis, require an immediate airway. However, patients who are awake can be considered for awake intubation. Awake intubation provides a method for managing a difficult airway without suppressing the patient's respirations or airway reflexes (Langeron et al. 2006). In most emergency situations, it is unlikely to be a realistic option; however, it is a technique that surgeons providing emergency care should be familiar with. The basic method consists of:

1. Local anesthetic applied via an atomizer or nebulizer to blunt the airway reflexes
2. Preoxygenation with a nonrebreather mask followed by nasal cannula
3. Light sedation

Box 6.2 Patients with a high suspicion for difficult airway
- Massive airway or facial trauma
- Obesity
- Short or thick neck
- Inability to completely visualize posterior oropharynx

4. Intubation with an endotracheal tube or bougie (Bailenson et al. 1967).

Most emergency situations, however, do not allow for the use of awake intubation and instead the use of sedation and muscle relaxants is essential. Rapid sequence intubation (RSI) can be utilized in most emergency situations requiring endotracheal intubation, but caution must be used.

Rapid sequence intubation

RSI is well-established as the preferred method of providing a secure and expedient airway in the emergency (yet somewhat controlled) setting. At its core, the goal of RSI is to render the patient unconscious and paralyzed in a rapid fashion, thus eliminating the risk of vomiting and aspiration. As previously mentioned, RSI is not the method of choice in patients with a suspected difficult airway or for those who are in extremis and not breathing. The basic method consists of:

1. Preoxygenation with high-flow oxygen preferably with little or no positive pressure ventilation
2. Premedication with lidocaine to prevent dysrhythmias, opioid analgesics, atropine for the prevention of bradycardia, and defasciculating agents
3. Induction
4. Intubation

Commonly used induction agents include ketamine, etomidate, propofol, and midazolam. The authors' preference is to use etomidate in most trauma or critically ill surgical patients due to its rapid onset, short duration, and minimal effect on hemodynamics when compared with other agents. Neuromuscular blockage is achieved using either depolarizing or nondepolarizing agents such as succinylcholine and rocuronium, respectively. Advantages of succinylcholine include rapid onset and short duration of effect. Succinylcholine should not be used in crush injuries, burns, or in patients at risk of hyperkalemia (Reynolds & Heffner 2005).

Anesthesiologists and nurse anesthetists in the emergency department

High-volume trauma centers and busy urban emergency departments may have diverse staffing, including trauma surgeons, emergency department physicians, and mid-level providers who often have additional training in emergency care. The role of anesthesiologists and nurse anesthetists can be complimentary in this setting, allowing for surgical and medical providers to focus on the overall care of the injured or critically ill patient while the airway is obtained by practitioners with the highest level of training in that area. While little data exist that demonstrate a direct improvement in outcomes when anesthesiologists or nurse anesthetists provide airway support, it is known that the risk of complications increases with the number of attempts at intubation. Similarly, it has been shown that, regardless of professional training, providers with the most experience in obtaining difficult airways have the greatest success. Thus, the availability of highly trained and experienced providers cannot be underestimated (Hartmannsgruber et al. 2000).

Use of assisted airway management in the emergency department

As previously mentioned, the patient in extremis or in respiratory failure requires rapid and effective airway control. Knowledge and skill with common airway adjuncts are essential in these situations. Devices such as the bougie, LMA (**Figure 6.1**), GlideScope (**Figure 6.2**), or fiberoptic scope should be readily available and ready for use at any time. It is prudent to employ adjuncts as early as possible after failed intubation. One failed attempt by an experienced provider should prompt consideration of the use of any of the adjuncts mentioned above. Surgeons and all those who provide care in the emergency department should familiarize themselves with the indications and correct use of the adjuncts available to them. The bougie stylet is readily available in most emergency departments and is easy to use. Disadvantages of bougies include a risk of blind insertion, which can result in oropharyngeal or bronchial trauma. Video laryngoscopes (e.g. GlideScope) and fiberoptic scopes provide the advantage of direct visualization of the vocal cords but can be similarly limited by blood or secretions in the airway. Other disadvantages to video-assisted devices include cost and maintenance and, in some instances, increased time to intubation. Supraglottic devices such as the LMA or Combitube

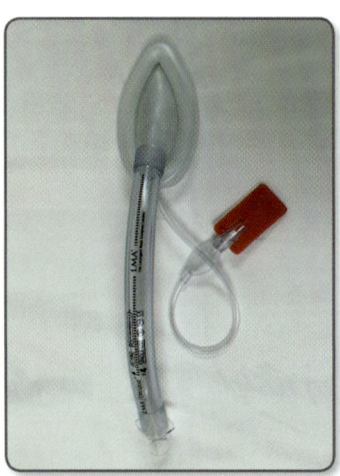

Figure 6.1 Laryngeal mask airway (LMA).

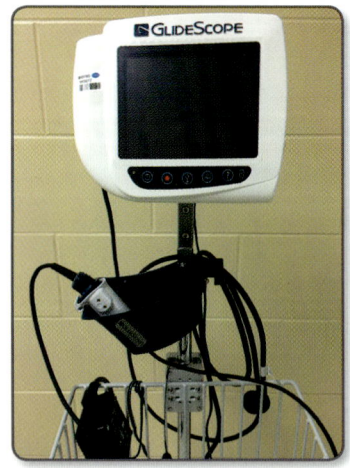

Figure 6.2 GlideScope video laryngoscope.

are easy to place and require minimal manipulation of the cervical spine when immobilization is necessary. Disadvantages include lower oxygen delivery and poor ventilation when compared with endotracheal intubation, as well as a higher risk of dislodgement and aspiration (Marco & Marco 2008).

Failed intubation, complications, and management

Even experienced and skilled providers will encounter difficulty and occasionally fail to successfully obtain endotracheal intubation. When oral or nasal intubation fails, it falls upon the surgeon in the emergency department to decide to cease further attempts and perform a cricothyroidotomy or tracheostomy instead. This decision must be made quickly, definitively, and acted upon immediately. This is essential to ensure a good outcome, as the patient is almost certainly hypoxic and often obtunded. In addition to having the proper instruments and equipment readily available, knowledge of the steps involved in either procedure is essential.

In the most desperate airway emergencies, the procedure of choice is cricothyroidotomy. This procedure is simple, fast, and effective, and it can also be performed with fewer instruments. After routine skin preparation and the application of local anesthetic, the operative steps are as follows:

1. With the neck in as much extension as possible, grasp the thyroid cartilage and palpate the cricothyroid membrane (**Figure 6.3**)
2. Using a number 15 scalpel, make a 2-cm transverse or vertical incision and carry it down to the cricothyroid membrane
3. Incise the cricothyroid membrane and turn the blade to create a space large enough to pass an endotracheal or 8-mm tracheostomy tube

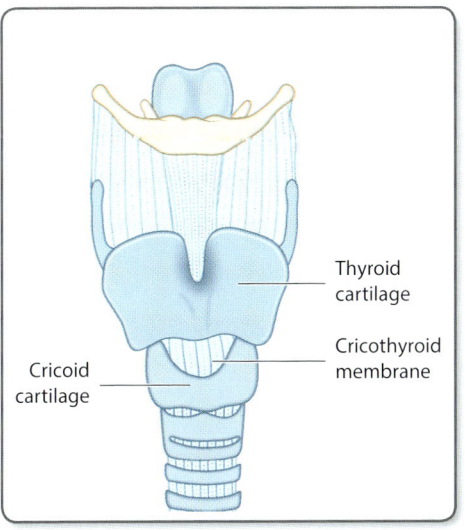

Figure 6.3 Trachea with landmarks for performing a cricothyroidotomy.

Thyroid cartilage

Cricothyroid membrane

Cricoid cartilage

4. Alternatively, a hemostat or tonsil can be used to open the trachea after it is incised allowing for passage of a tube (**Figure 6.4**)
5. Confirm the correct placement by looking for equal chest rise and auscultate for equal air entry, and return of end-tidal CO_2
6. Secure the airway using nylon sutures

Tracheostomy can also be performed in the emergency department but requires more preparation, equipment, and time. Therefore, tracheostomy may not be ideal for patients in extremis. While it can be performed under local anesthesia, the use of sedation is encouraged. After skin preparation, the operative steps are as follows:

1. With the neck in as much extension as possible, palpate the cricoid cartilage and identify the first and second tracheal rings inferior to the cricoid cartilage (**Figure 6.5**)
2. Using a number 15 scalpel, make a 3–4-cm transverse incision at the level of the second tracheal ring and carry the incision down to the platysma, carefully obtaining hemostasis

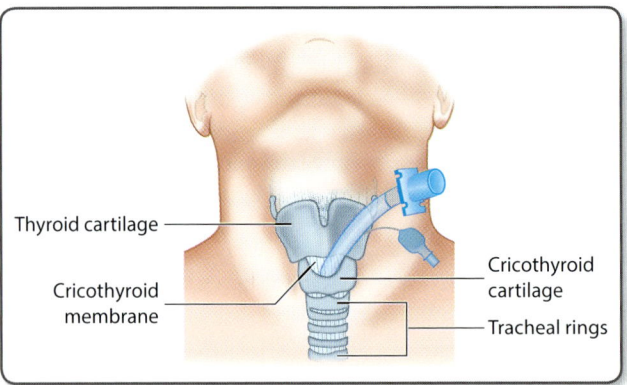

Thyroid cartilage

Cricothyroid membrane

Cricothyroid cartilage

Tracheal rings

Figure 6.4 Endotracheal tube in place following an emergency cricothyroidotomy.

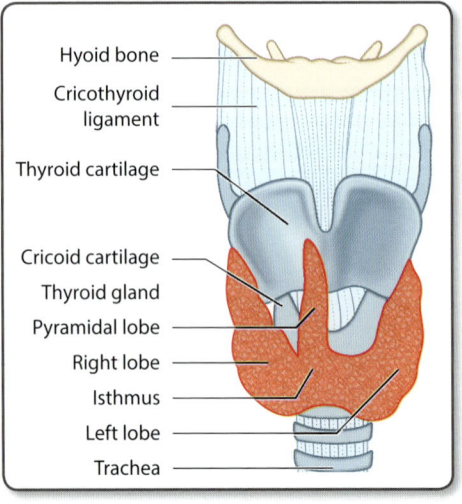

Hyoid bone
Cricothyroid ligament
Thyroid cartilage
Cricoid cartilage
Thyroid gland
Pyramidal lobe
Right lobe
Isthmus
Left lobe
Trachea

Figure 6.5 Trachea with landmarks for performing a tracheostomy.

3. Using electrocautery, divide the platysma to expose the strap muscles. Place a retractor to further visualize the strap muscles and separate them in the midline using electrocautery

4. Carefully avoid the isthmus of the thyroid, which often lies over the third tracheal ring. Injury to the isthmus can cause bleeding that can be difficult and time-consuming to control

5. The isthmus can be retracted cephalad or caudad to expose the second tracheal ring, which can be further cleared of connective tissue

6. If time allows, place stay sutures laterally through the ring that will be divided to open the trachea. These are left long and secured to the skin. Stay sutures facilitate exposure and replacement of the tracheostomy tube if it should be removed or fall out

7. Ensure excellent hemostasis before opening the trachea

8. Divide the second tracheal ring in the midline with a vertical incision using a scalpel. Make horizontal incisions in the membranes above and below this ring, creating flaps on either side of the vertical incision that divided the ring (**Figure 6.6**)

9. Using a tracheal spreader, dilate the defect in the trachea and insert an 8 mm tracheostomy tube. Ensure adequate placement by confirming equal chest rise, auscultation, and return of end-tidal CO_2 (**Figure 6.7**)

10. Secure the tracheostomy tube to the skin using nylon sutures. Use cotton tapes or tracheostomy straps to further secure the airway around the patient's neck (Scott-Conner 2002)

An emergency airway algorithm that can be broadly applied in the care of trauma or critically ill surgical patients in the emergency department is shown in **Figure 6.8**.

Conclusion

Management of the acute airway in the emergency department can be challenging. In any airway emergency, adherence to a management algorithm that is tailored to the practices of the emergency team is crucial. Guidelines for steps to follow in an airway emergency are

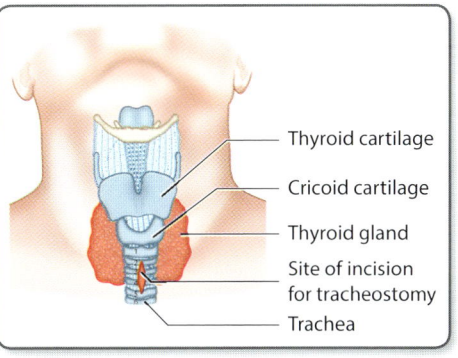

Figure 6.6 Trachea with site of incision for tracheostomy.

Thyroid cartilage

Cricoid cartilage

Thyroid gland

Site of incision for tracheostomy

Trachea

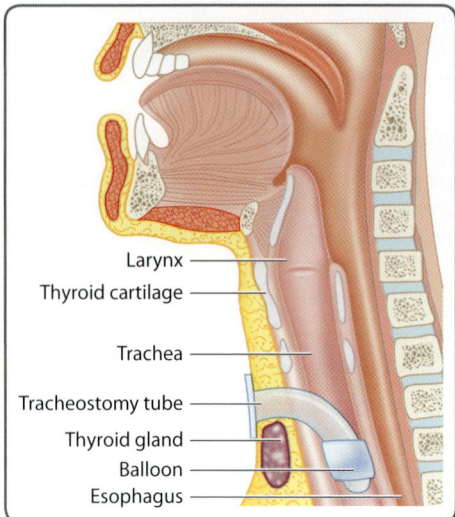

Figure 6.7 Sagittal view of trachea.

Larynx
Thyroid cartilage
Trachea
Tracheostomy tube
Thyroid gland
Balloon
Esophagus

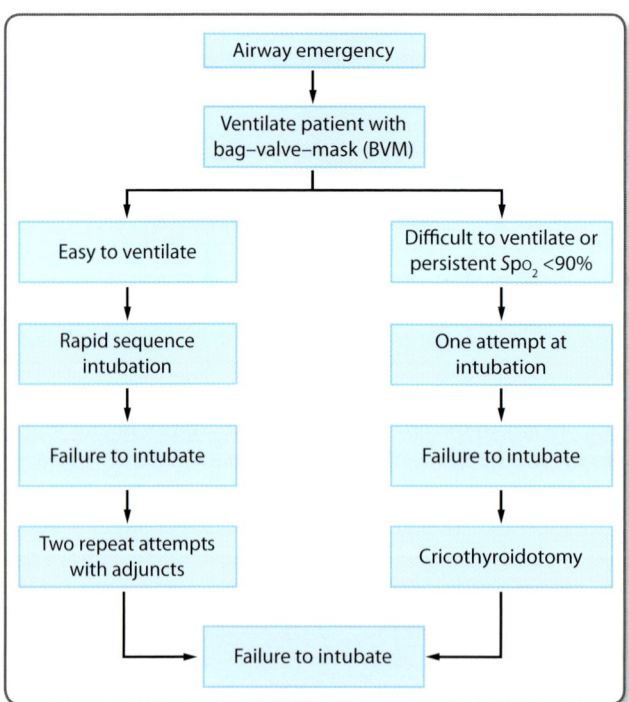

Figure 6.8 Algorithm for dealing with an airway emergency.

Airway emergency

Ventilate patient with bag–valve–mask (BVM)

Easy to ventilate

Difficult to ventilate or persistent Spo_2 <90%

Rapid sequence intubation

One attempt at intubation

Failure to intubate

Failure to intubate

Two repeat attempts with adjuncts

Cricothyroidotomy

Failure to intubate

essential to avoid confusion and disorder in a situation that can easily become life threatening. Equally important is a broad knowledge of airway adjuncts, competences in their use, and knowing when to perform a surgical airway. As with any procedure, the ease of and experience with the steps involved will increase the chances of success and a good patient outcome.

References

Bailenson G, Turbin J, Berman R. Awake intubation: indications and technique. Anesth Prog 1967; 14:272–278.

Berlac P, Hyldmo PK, Kongstad P, et al; Scandinavian Society for Anesthesiology and Intensive Care Medicine. Pre-hospital airway management: guidelines from a task force from the Scandinavian Society for Anaesthesiology and Intensive Care Medicine. Acta Anaesthesiol Scand 2008; 52:897–907.

Hartmannsgruber MW, Gabrielli A, Layon AJ, Rosenbaum SH. The traumatic airway: the anesthesiologist's role in the emergency room. Int Anesthesiol Clin 2000; 38:87–104.

Langeron O, Amour J, Vivien B, Aubrun F. Clinical review: management of difficult airways. Crit Care 2006; 10:243.

Marco CA, Marco AP. Airway adjuncts. Emerg Med Clin North Am 2008; 26: 1015–1027.

Reynolds SF, Heffner J. Airway management of the critically ill patient: rapid-sequence intubation. Chest 2005; 127:1397–1412.

Scott-Conner CEH. Chassin's operative strategy in general surgery: an expositive atlas. New York: Springer, 2002.

7

Equipment

Jerome W Thompson

Introduction

Bag mask airway is one of the oldest and yet least well-applied techniques for maintaining an airway. For decades this was the standard method of administering anesthesia. When used properly in an airway emergency, it can maintain an airway indefinitely. During cardiac arrests or 'codes,' conditions and available equipment are often far from ideal. Many airway issues can go wrong. An oral airway or trumpet is not in use or it is the wrong size, the mask-bag valve is not adjusted properly (**Figure 7.1**), there is neither enough head extension nor is a tight enough fit or seal of the mask obtained. Maintaining an airway is truly an underappreciated skill, frequently overlooked in the training of a surgeon.

First, there must be a posterior rotation of the head, tilting the vertex back and down. This must then be coupled with a jaw thrust by pushing the tip of the chin down to open the mouth and an anterior dislocation of the jaw joint with the fingers from behind, to bring the jaw and tongue forward to open the airway and allow insertion of an oral airway (**Figure 7.2**). There are multiple sizes of masks to choose from, ranging from neonate to large adult. The seal can frequently be adjusted with a syringe (**Figure 7.3**). The mask can be held with one or two hands, depending on the resources and circumstances prevailing at the time. There are multiple sizes, and two different styles, of plastic oral airways and rubber trumpets (**Figure 7.4**). The correct technique for inserting an airway is to first put it in upside down against the palate and then to rotate it clockwise, pushing it posteriorly behind the tongue, separating the tongue from the posterior pharyngeal wall. If the jaws are locked together, one or two nasal trumpets can be inserted to provide an

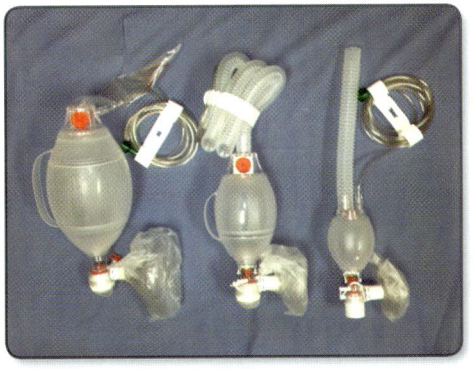

Figure 7.1 Assorted sizes of Ambu bags and masks from infant (right) to adult (left).

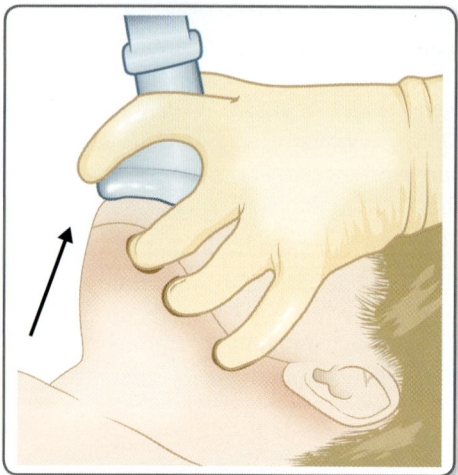

Figure 7.2 Hand position and head rotation for proper mask ventilation.

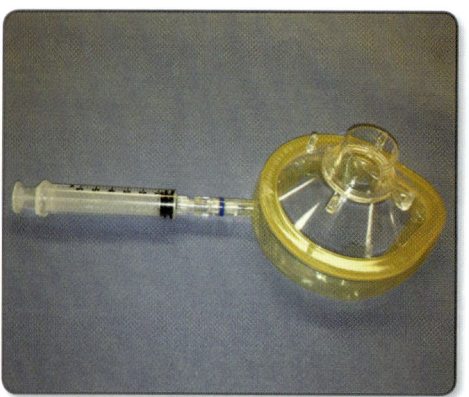

Figure 7.3 Syringe inflation of mask cuff for proper fit and air seal.

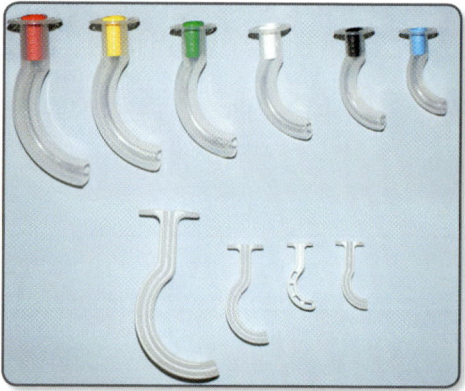

Figure 7.4 Several types and sizes of oral airways.

airway past the tongue until the jaw relaxes. One of the hazards of bag mask ventilation is inadvertent inflation of the stomach, which could then push up against the diaphragm and make effective ventilation difficult. The Sellick maneuver (pressing on the cricoid while bagging the patient) can be performed to prevent air from going into the upper esophagus and subsequently into the stomach.

Laryngoscopes

Otolaryngologic scopes

The most striking difference between otolaryngologic laryngoscopes and others is that they are straight and can only be inserted when the head and neck are extended posterior or back. The first were introduced by Jackson and Hollinger, then came Dedo scopes that were suspended from gallows or held by hand. These are still in use today, 90 years later. Modern scopes in use today use fiberoptic light carriers or prisms rather than bulbs (**Figure 7.5**), and the suspension apparatus are far more sophisticated (**Figure 7.6**). The intensity of illumination is from a 300-W source, which is 10 times than that of a battery-powered anesthesia scope. With these, there are no shadows in the pharynx or larynx, which makes intubation significantly easier. Some of these scopes are completely enclosed and the metal darkened so that they can reduce laser reflections and allow passage of instruments so as to prevent damage to adjacent tissue. The suspension system allows the clinician to work on a difficult laryngeal lesion with two hands direct vision, a microscope or video telescopes. There are many different sizes available and adjustable laryngoscopes to accommodate any shape or size of airway. Optic telescopic laryngoscopes, which can be connected to a TV camera, have even been made for difficult intubation (**Figure 7.7**).

Anesthesia scopes

Macintosh blades are one of the oldest types of blade and come in numerous sizes. They are battery powered and thus have limited intensity. They are curved so that they will arch around the tongue and rest in the vallecula. The head must be flexed up on a lift or pillow, and

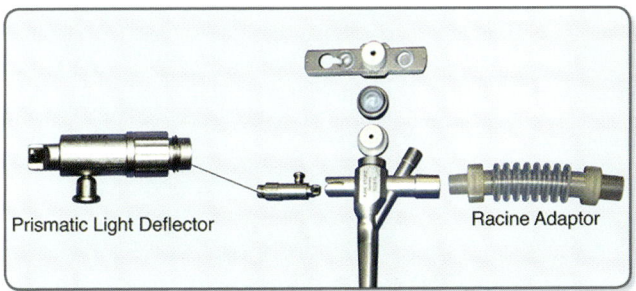

Figure 7.5 Proper Storz bronchoscope assembly. ©2014 Photo Courtesy of Karl Storz Endoscopy-America, Inc.

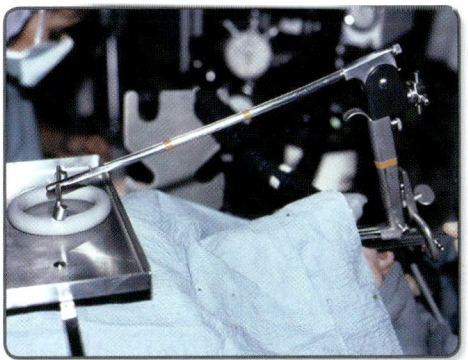

Figure 7.6 Modern Storz laryngeal suspension.

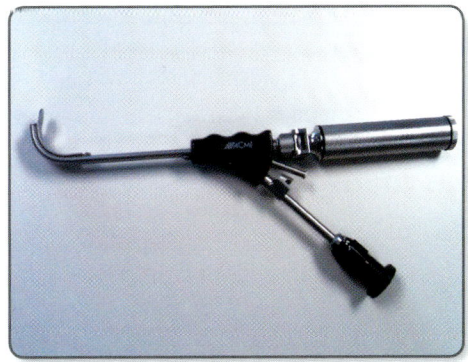

Figure 7.7 Bullard telescopic laryngoscope.

the blade must lift the tongue up, and go into the vallecula to visualize the larynx (**Figure 7.8**). The handle must be lifted forward and upward at a 45° angle to the axis of the patient (**Figure 7.9**).

Miller blades are straight and go into the larynx, with the head extended and the handle lifted straight up at a 90° angle to the axis of the patient (**Figure 7.10**). Both blades are used in conjunction with an endotracheal tube with a soft metal stylet that allows the user to shape the endotracheal tube with a bend to go around a corner. Both types of blade can be used with a pair of McGill forceps to guide the endotracheal tube into the larynx.

The GlideScope or distal chip video laryngoscope is a significant advancement in the management of difficult airways (**Figure 7.11**). These scopes place a single chip TV camera at the end of a disposable plastic Macintosh laryngoscope blade, which allows the intubator to see the larynx on an adjacent TV screen in many of the most difficult

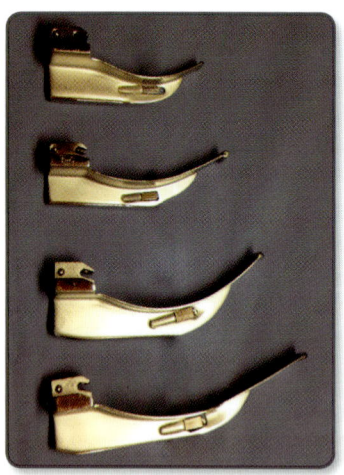

Figure 7.8 Assorted Macintosh laryngoscope blades.

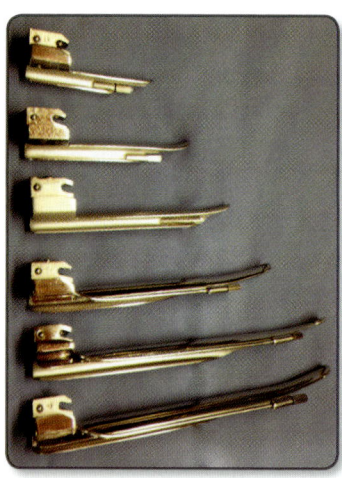

Figure 7.10 Assorted Miller laryngoscope blades.

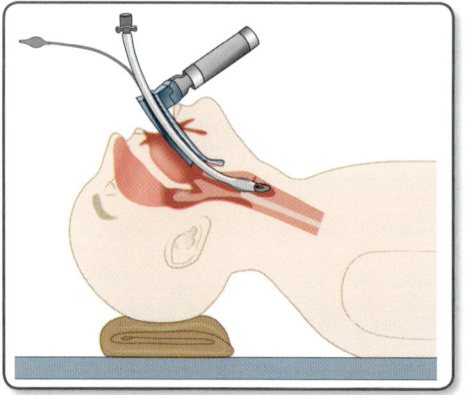

Figure 7.9 Intubation technique with a Macintosh blade.

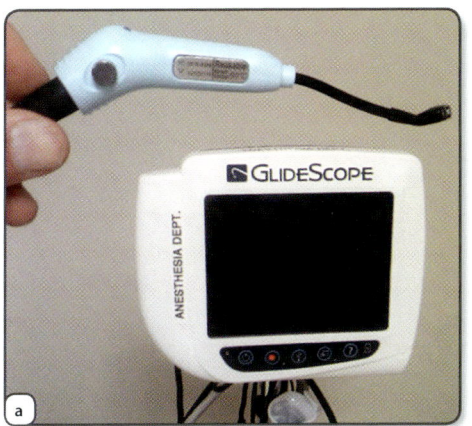 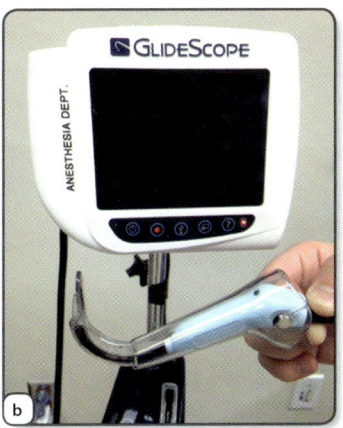

Figure 7.11 (a) GlideScope screen and probe. (b) Probe inserted into plastic Macintosh blade handle.

of airways. This device has made many difficult airways more easily managed.

Outside the hospital environment, up to 25% of endotracheal tubes are misplaced and 13% fail (Denninghoff et al. 2000). There are four basic errors that lead to failed intubation.

1. A rushed laryngoscopy with a poor choice—or no choice at all—of the size or type of laryngoscope or endotracheal tube. Suction may also not be available or working
2. Failure to have a backup plan for maintaining the airway intubation not be possible. Alternative medications for relaxation or paralysis need to have been considered at the outset
3. Poor tongue control. Otolaryngologic scopes keep the tongue to the left of the scope, while Miller and MacIntosh blades compress the tongue into the midline and thus into the floor of the mouth
4. Poor position of the head or scope. The MacIntosh blade is designed to go into the vallecula, while the Miller and most otolaryngologic blades can go either into the vallecula or under the epiglottis and directly into the larynx.

Practice using mannequins and direct supervision by senior practitioners of many early intubations should be a mandated part of every surgeon's training. The most common complications of intubation are loosened or broken teeth, bleeding from the tongue, pharynx, larynx, or laryngeal edema from repeated blunt trauma.

The laryngeal mask airway

The laryngeal mask airway is a device that is inserted into the mouth and down to cover the larynx with a small pharyngeal mask that is then inflated and connected to a bag or anesthesia circuit (**Figure 7.12**). They have been very effective in difficult airway cases, such as patients with Pierre Robin syndrome or other patients presenting with micrognathia, and come in many different sizes. They also eliminate

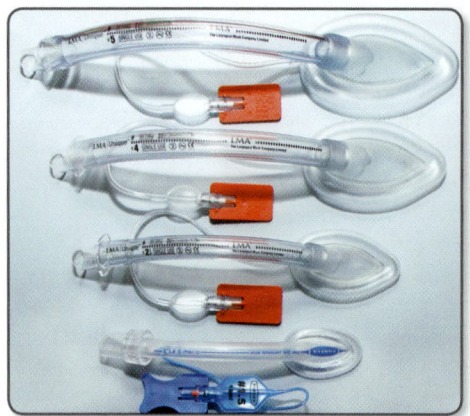

Figure 7.12 Assorted sizes of laryngeal mask airway.

the need to instrument the larynx or subglottic airway in brief cases and thus eliminate the risk of traumatic subglottic or laryngeal edema. The distal baffles in the mask can be cut out, thus allowing the passage at a later stage of flexible fiberoptic scopes with endotracheal tubes. They do, however, tend to become dislodged with high positive pressure or excessive movement of the head or neck.

Emergent airways

Paramedics in the field have used esophageal airways to establish a functional airway in a rescue situation. These are useful because it is easier to pass a tube into the larger esophagus than the smaller larynx. These tubes take advantage of this fact by intentionally allowing for the intubation of the esophagus and then inflation of a balloon there. There is a second passage that opens at approximately the level of the larynx for ventilation and a second balloon above that opening to seal the pharynx. Such devices are very effective in the hands of those not trained to intubate the larynx.

Flexible fiberoptic endoscopes

Large diameter flexible fiberoptic scopes were originally designed for gastrointestinal diagnostic uses. They have been modified from their original form to a shorter and smaller fiber diameter so that they may pass through the nose, an endotracheal tube or bronchus. They can be used for difficult intubations by allowing the physician to slide the endotracheal tube over the smaller flexible fiberoptic scope and then pass both devices through the nose and into the larynx and trachea. The tube is advanced over the scope as a tube-guide into the airway in difficult situations where the mouth cannot be opened. This can be combined with a regular Macintosh blade to get past the tongue and facilitate intubation.

Rigid bronchoscopes have been used for over a hundred years to secure difficult airways. They must be passed through a laryngoscope and then into the airway. These scopes offer the added advantage of allowing the ventilation of the patient as well as the removal of tumors and foreign bodies, unlike flexible bronchoscopes. They can be illuminated by prisms or by fiberoptic light carriers. There are two basic types of bronchoscopes: those that are open and those that are sealed (telescopic). Telescopic scopes can be fitted with a TV camera and the bronchi displayed on a widescreen TV. An enormous variety of instruments may be passed through these scopes, such as biopsy forceps, peanut grasping forceps, and forceps with teeth to remove food foreign bodies such as meat. The distal end of the bronchoscope has side ports to allow the ventilation of the opposite bronchus, while the tip of the scope is in the other. There are also suction ports for clearing secretions and lavaging for culture and sensitivity.

Lasers

There are numerous types of lasers: CO_2 fiber, KTP (potassium titanyl phosphate) YAG lasers, and Argon lasers to name but a few commonly used in surgery. Each has a specific wavelength and tissue destruction characteristic. The CO_2 laser tends to be favored for laryngeal tumor work. New, flexible CO_2 fibers allow work in small areas that are not in the direct line of sight (**Figure 7.13**). Lasers can destroy tumors or structures that obstruct the airway, thus making them manageable. However, all lasers pose a hazard of inadvertent tissue destruction, and the CO_2 laser is also a potential fire hazard. Great care must be exercised with lasers due to the risk of eye damage, and special wavelength-specific eyewear must be used at all times for staff and patients. Wet protective sponges should be placed over the patient's eyes before the CO_2 procedure begins. Because of the high heat generated and the presence of fuel (fat, drapes, sponges) and oxygen, there is a certain fire risk. Laser fires have been reported, and precautions such as wet towels and large syringes full of water must be available. Laser-resistant

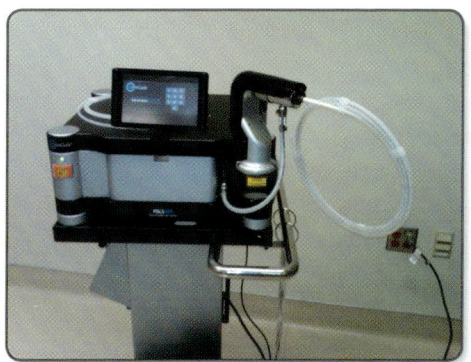

Figure 7.13 Flexible fiberoptic CO_2 laser.

endotracheal tubes are available, but studies show that all of them can be ignited by repeated 'hits' with the laser. Training is vital to ensure that practitioners can manage such situations should they occur. Fire during laryngoscopy and bronchoscopy is probably the most common scenario due to the need to ventilate the patient with oxygen. One study (Thompson et al. 1998) showed that a CO_2 laser was safe in an oxygen atmosphere of <45% with anesthetic gases. Should fire ignite in the airway, then the endotracheal tube should be removed, or the bronchoscope removed, O_2 delivery should be stopped, water applied to the field, and the patient mask ventilated. Patients who suffer burns to the airway do remarkably well, and the application of antibiotics, steroids, and a cool mist for about 10 days usually helps alleviate the damage sustained.

Conclusion

There have been major leaps of progress in the equipment used to manage the airway over the past 3,000 years. Frequently, wars have stimulated advancement but now it is the steady advance of technology in the past 50 years that is driving the rapid (sometimes daily) improvement in the equipment we have available to secure and trial the airway. Physicians must be constantly receptive to new ideas and treatment protocols – the future is approaching more rapidly than we think.

References

Denninghoff KR, Griffin MJ, Bartolucci AA, et al. Emergent endotracheal intubation and mortality in traumatic brain injury. West J Emerg Med 2000; 9:184–189.
Thompson JW, Colin W, Snowden T, et al. Fire in the operating room during tracheostomy. South Med J 1998;91:243-247.

8

Pediatric airway management part 1: overview and congenital anomalies

Jennifer McLevy, Jerome W Thompson, Rose Mary S Stocks

Introduction

The management of the pediatric airway has several unique and striking features that differentiate it from the management of the adult airway. Not only are there key anatomical and physiological differences, but these differences also change as the child grows from neonate to infant, from infant to child, and from child to adolescent. The equipment to adequately assess and manage the pediatric airway also reflects the changing needs of the patients as they grow.

Anatomy and physiology

There are three key anatomical sites that differentiate the management of a pediatric airway from that of an adult airway.

Tongue

The tongue lies in contact with both the hard and soft palates during infancy. It is proportionately larger than the remainder of the oral cavity. Its positioning and redundancy increase the risk of airway obstruction in the neonate. The discrepancy in positioning and redundancy of the tongue erode as the child ages from 1 to 10 years old.

Larynx

There are three key differentiating components of the pediatric larynx. The first key component is the overall position of the larynx. In a premature neonate, the larynx is positioned the most cephalic, at the level of the third cervical vertebra (C3) (Cote et al. 2013). The larynx is located at C3–4 in a term neonate and migrates over the next 10–12 years to reach the adult position. The cephalic position of the larynx in the premature and term infants, in conjunction with the concurrent tongue position, contributes to rendering the infant an obligate nasal breather for the first few months of life. The second key component is the shape and position of the epiglottis. In the infant, the epiglottis is Ω shaped and narrower than that of the adult. The final component is the angle of the vocal folds. Unlike the adult, where the vocal fold axis is perpendicular to the trachea, the anterior insertion of the vocal folds is more caudal than the posterior insertion (Cote et al. 2013).

Subglottis

The airway of the infant is more cone shaped than that of the adult, and the narrowest portion of the infant airway is the cricoid cartilage (**Figure 8.1**). The infant cricoid has a diameter of 4–5 mm, and, being the only complete ring in the airway, it is not able to be distended. The cricoid is lined by pseudostratified columnar epithelium, and pressure to this nondistensible site in the form of an overly tight endotracheal tube (ETT), for example, may create reactive edema and a subsequent decrease in lumen diameter. Airway resistance is roughly derived from Poiseuille's law: R is proportional to $1/r^4$, where R is the resistance and r is the radius (Cote et al. 2013). Therefore, a 1 mm reduction in a 4 mm infant airway can produce a 75% increase in airway resistance (Cote et al. 2013). The subglottis grows rapidly from birth to 2 years of age and then linearly from 2 to 10–12 years of age. The cricoid and thyroid cartilages then reach the adult proportions. Of note, the cricothyroid membrane in children from <3–4 years old is minute, rendering needle cricothyrotomy very difficult and surgical cricothyrotomy impossible. Surgical cricothyrotomy is contraindicated until the patient is more than 10–12 years old.

The key physiologic properties that differentiate pediatric from adult airway management involve oxygen consumption, functional residual capacity (FRC), and the location of greatest airway resistance. The basal oxygen consumption rate of a full-term neonate is roughly two times that of an adult, while in case of a premature infant it is three times that of an adult (Cote et al. 2013). The FRC of the child is also proportionately smaller than that of the adult. The increased thoracic and lung compliance of the infant greatly contributes to this reduction in FRC. In the infant, the location of the greatest airway resistance is the tracheobronchial tree, while in the adult, it is in the nasal passage. The clinical significance of these physiologic differences is that oxygen desaturation is more rapid and dynamic airway collapse is far more likely in children (Cote et al. 2013) (**Figure 8.2**). Airway intervention

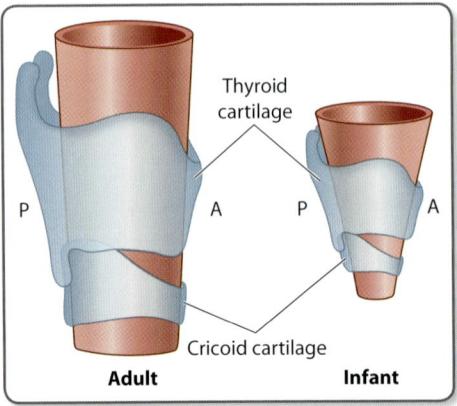

Figure 8.1 Configuration of the larynx of an adult (a) and an infant (b). Notice that both larynxes are somewhat funnel-shaped, but this shape is exaggerated in infants and toddlers. The adult laryngeal structures are of such a size that most endotracheal tubes (ETTs) pass easily into the trachea. In infants and toddlers, it is common for the ETT to pass easily through the vocal cords but to become snug at the level of the nondistensible cricoid cartilage. Concern for causing edema at this point resulted in the classic teaching that uncuffed ETTs should be used in young children (A, anterior; P, posterior). With permission from Cote CJ, Lerman J, Anderson BJ. A practice of anesthesia for infants and children, 5th edn. Philadelphia, PA: Saunders, 2013:237–276.

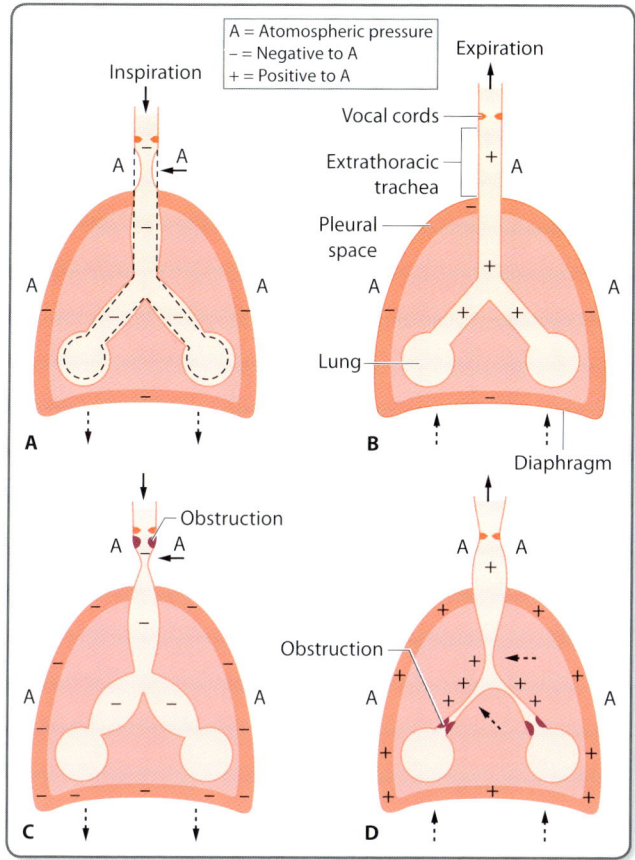

Figure 8.2 (a) With descent of the diaphragm and contraction of the intercostal muscles, a greater negative intrathoracic pressure relative to intraluminal and atmospheric pressure is developed. The net result is longitudinal stretching of the larynx and trachea, dilatation of the intrathoracic trachea and bronchi, movement of air into the lungs, and some dynamic collapse of the extrathoracic trachea (arrow). The dynamic collapse is due to the highly compliant trachea and the negative intraluminal pressure in relation to atmospheric pressure. (b) The normal sequence of events at end expiration is a slight negative intrapleural pressure stenting the airways open. In infants, the highly compliant chest does not provide the support required; therefore, airway closure occurs with each breath. Intraluminal pressures are slightly positive in relation to atmospheric pressure, with the result that air is forced out of the lungs. (c) Obstructed extrathoracic airway. Notice the severe dynamic collapse of the extrathoracic trachea below the level of obstruction. This collapse is greatest at the thoracic inlet, where the largest pressure gradient exists between negative intratracheal pressure and atmospheric pressure (arrow). (Extrathoracic upper airway obstruction is characterized by inspiratory stridor.) (d) Obstructed intrathoracic trachea or airways. Notice that breathing against an obstructed lower airway (e.g. bronchiolitis, asthma) results in greater positive intrathoracic pressures, with dynamic collapse of the intrathoracic airways [prolonged expiration or wheezing (arrows)]. With permission from Cote CJ, Lerman J, Anderson BJ. A practice of anesthesia for infants and children, 5th edn. Philadelphia, PA: Saunders, 2013:237–276.

must therefore be more rapid in children, and keeping a child in airway distress calm is of paramount importance to avoid airway collapse.

Pediatric instruments and equipment

Endoscopy

Endoscopy may be performed for both diagnostic and therapeutic purposes. Diagnostically, endoscopy may be used to evaluate structures, gather cultures, and obtain biopsies. The therapeutic indications include foreign body or mucous plug removal, neoplastic intervention, cyst removal, airway dilation, and emergently obtaining an airway in an obstructing patient (Bluestone et al. 2003).

Flexible fiberoptic nasopharyngoscopy

The flexible fiberoptic nasopharyngoscope may be used to evaluate the anatomy and function of the nasal cavity, nasopharynx, oropharynx, and larynx of the awake patient in all age groups. As neonates and infants are more prone to rapid desaturation and laryngospasm, special care must be taken to perform the flexible nasolaryngoscopy in a monitored setting with meticulous technique. Defogging of the tip and lubrication of the endoscope are recommended. Some practitioners apply a topical anesthetic (e.g. 2% lidocaine) and/or decongestant (e.g. oxymetazoline) to the nasal cavities prior to commencing the procedure. The diameter of the nasopharyngoscopes ranges from 1.9 to 6 mm, and the lengths come in pediatric to adult sizes. A video tower may be used in conjunction with the endoscope to project the image, record the examination, and print off images for further review after the procedure.

Direct laryngoscopy

Direct laryngoscopy and bronchoscopy should be performed in an operating room or similarly monitored setting. The anesthesia laryngoscopes may be used for intubation purposes. The straight (Miller) blade is narrower and may be used to lift the epiglottis, allowing direct visualization of the vocal folds. The straight blade is often used in children from 2 years old and younger. The curved (Macintosh) blade is advanced into the vallecula and is frequently employed in older children and adults. There are three main types of otolaryngology laryngoscopes—the standard, the subglottic, and the anterior commissure laryngoscope—which typically use a fiberoptic light carrier to attach to a xenon light source (Bluestone et al. 2003). After placing a tooth guard, the laryngoscope is advanced into the vallecula for the initial assessment. When placed into suspension, documentation of the laryngoscopy may be done by attaching a rod telescope to a camera system. Additionally, a binocular microscope, with a 400 mm lens, may be used to perform microsurgical procedures.

Bronchoscopy

Both rigid and flexible bronchoscopes are available. A major benefit of using a rigid bronchoscope is that it has a port to provide concurrent ventilation. In the setting of an emergency with difficult intubation, the rigid bronchoscope provides excellent visualization to obtain the airway while offering ventilation. In extreme circumstances, an emergency tracheostomy may be performed while the airway is maintained with the rigid bronchoscope. Rigid bronchoscopes come in a variety of diameters and lengths. Storz pediatric rigid bronchoscopes are available in the following sizes according to the child's age group (Bluestone et al. 2003) (**Figure 8.3**):

- Premature infants and neonates: 2.5–3.5 diameter, 20 cm length
- Infants: 3.0–4.0 diameter, 26 cm length
- Older children: 3.5–6.0 diameter, 30 cm length

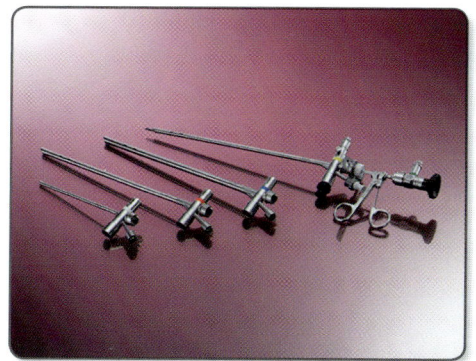

Figure 8.3 Storz pediatric bronchoscopes. ©2014 Photo courtesy of Karl Storz Endoscopy-America, Inc.

The rod telescopes, which are usually used in conjunction with the bronchoscope, come in 0°, 30°, and 70° options. Most commonly, the 0° telescope is employed during bronchoscopy. After placing the tooth guard, the patient is positioned with his/her head extended and the neck flexed, often with a shoulder roll in place. Frequently, a laryngoscope is employed initially to introduce the bronchoscope. The bronchoscope is rotated 90° to pass between the vocal folds. Once in position, the bronchoscope is advanced between the thumb and the forefinger of the left hand. With the rod attached to a camera system, the procedure may be visualized and documented more easily. In the lumen of the tracheobronchial tree, other optic instruments may be used to perform procedures such as foreign body removal or to obtain biopsies. The main risks associated with rigid endoscopy include dental damage, arytenoid dislocation, laryngospasm, and airway perforation. The complication rate is approximately 2–3% (Bluestone et al. 2003).

The flexible bronchoscope does not contain a side port for ventilation. In older children with a larger tracheal lumen, spontaneous ventilation is possible around the flexible bronchoscope while the patient is sedated. The flexible bronchoscope provides excellent visualization of more distal bronchial anatomy. In addition, an ETT may be passed over the flexible bronchoscope, thus allowing improved visualization during a difficult intubation.

Equipment

Airways

Oral and nasal airways are an excellent adjunct to bypass prolapsing structures, thereby assisting with supplemental oxygenation. Oral airways are used in the unconscious patient who lacks a gag reflex. The size is selected by using an oral airway that fits between the angle of the mouth and the tragus of the ear. If the oral airway is too small, it will not prevent the collapse of the base of the tongue, but if it is too large, an oral airway will produce an obstruction (American Heart Association 2005). Nasopharyngeal airways are used in the responsive patient. The size is selected by measuring from the tip of the nose to the ear tragus.

If the naris blanches after insertion, the airway is too large and must be downsized. Care must be taken to suction them frequently, so as to prevent obstruction by secretions.

Endotracheal tubes

The inner diameter (ID) size of the uncuffed pediatric ETT in children from 1 to 10 years old can be calculated using the following formula (American Heart Association 2005):

$$\text{Uncuffed ETT ID size} = (\text{Age in years}/4) + 4.$$

For a premature infant, the size is usually 2.5–3.0 mm ID; for a term infant it is usually a 3.0–3.5 mm ID; and for a 1-year-old it is usually 3.5–4.0 mm ID. To determine if the ID is appropriate, weight-based tidal volumes and an air leak between 10 and 20 cmH_2O of pressure are sought. The length is roughly calculated as three times the appropriate size tube (for the patient's age). Verification of placement is achieved by the following methods:

- Auscultation of equal bilateral breath sounds
- Carbon dioxide (CO_2) indicator (colorimetric)
- Capnography confirmation of CO_2 return
- Laryngoscopy revealing that the ETT is through the vocal folds
- Chest X-ray

As the cricoid ring has the smallest diameter of the pediatric airway, an uncuffed ETT is most commonly used. In patients with poor pulmonary compliance, high airway resistance, or an airway leak >20 cmH_2O, a cuffed ETT may be indicated. Care must be taken to keep the cuff inflation pressure <20 cmH_2O. The cuffed ETT ID size is calculated as follows (American Heart Association 2005):

$$\text{Cuffed ETT ID size} = (\text{Age in years}/4) + 3$$

Management of congenital anomalies

The management of congenital airway anomalies is determined by the anatomical site of the abnormality, its severity, and the timing of the presentation. The keys to determining the anomaly lie in the history of present illness and physical examination, assisted by endoscopy and necessary imaging. The following organs represent the most common congenital airway abnormalities that require the urgent attention of the surgeon, based on their anatomical locations.

Nose

Until the term neonate is 4–6 weeks old, they are obligate nasal breathers. Any condition causing complete nasal obstruction will result in respiratory distress, and ultimately, failure. Conditions such as frontonasal masses (e.g. dermoid, glioma and encephalocele) and neoplasms (e.g. hemangioma and lymphangioma, and rhabdomyosarcoma) are rare and do not frequently cause complete nasal obstruction in the neonate (Gnagi & Schraff 2013). If respiratory distress occurs, the airway should be established via intubation while the condition is assessed and the management plan is established. Nasolacrimal cysts and dacryocystoceles are usually unilateral and, therefore, respond well to conservative management.

The most common causes of neonatal bilateral nasal obstruction are choanal atresia and pyriform aperture stenosis. Choanal atresia is thought to arise from persistence of the buccopharyngeal membrane or failure of the oronasal membrane's rupture. The overall incidence of choanal atresia is 1 in 5000–8000 births with a 2:1 female:male ratio (Gnagi & Schraff 2013). About 25–30% are bilateral and 50% are associated with a syndrome, most commonly Coloboma, Heart disease, Atresia choanae, Retarded development of the central nervous system, Genitourinary hypoplasia, and Ear anomalies (CHARGE); (Gnagni & Schraff 2013). Bilateral choanal atresia typically presents as neonatal paradoxical cyanosis (cyanosis that improves with crying) and respiratory distress. Inability to pass a 6-French (Fr) catheter beyond 32 mm transnasally and nasal endoscopy revealing bilateral distal blind sacs are diagnostic (**Figure 8.4**) The CT scan reveals thickening of the vomer and the lateral wall of the nasal cavity and demonstrates what type of atresia is present (bony, membranous, mixed) (**Figure 8.5**). Initial management is to secure the airway with either an oral airway or McGovern nipple. If unsuccessful, intubation may be necessary to ensure a secure airway. Repair of bilateral choanal atresia typically occurs in the first 1–2 weeks of life. The surgical options include the following:

- Transnasal puncture
- Transpalatal repair
- Endoscopic transnasal approach with the consideration of the adjunctive use of postoperative stenting and laser

Unilateral choanal atresia repair is typically elective and performed in school-aged children. Congenital nasal pyriform aperture stenosis is far rarer and is thought to arise from the overgrowth of the maxillary

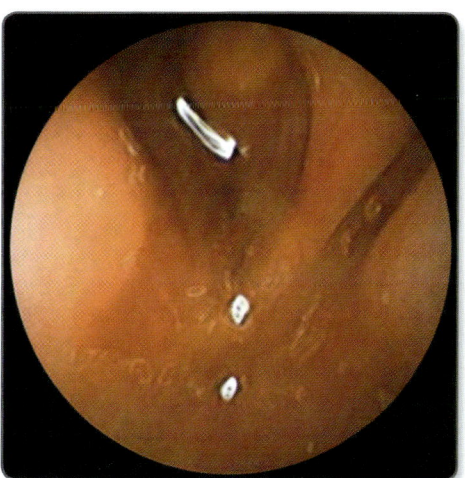

Figure 8.4 Nasal endoscopy revealing membranous occlusion of the posterior nasal cavity consistent with choanal atresia. With permission from Gnagi SH, Schraff SA. Nasal obstruction in newborns. Ped Clin North Am 2013; 60:903–922.

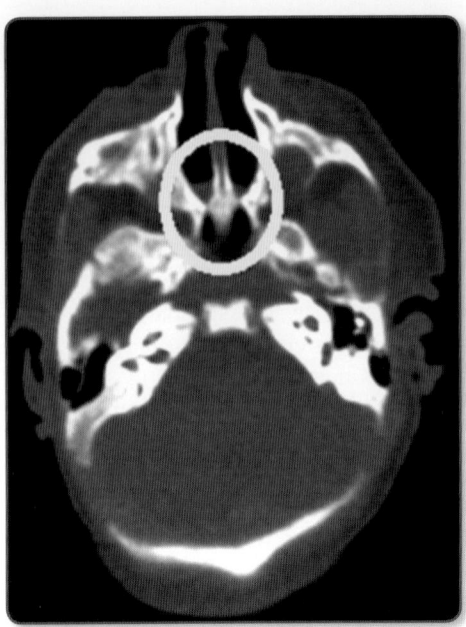

Figure 8.5 Axial computed tomography showing atretic choanae. Circle encompasses atresia at posterior nasal vault. With permission from Shah UK, Daniero JJ, Clary MS, et al. Low birth weight choanal atresia repair using image guidance. Int J Pediatr Otorhinolaryngol 2011; 75:1339.

nasal process. It may present as part of the holoprosencephaly sequence and also presents with neonatal paradoxical cyanosis and respiratory distress. Diagnostic keys include a single central incisor, an inability to pass a 6-Fr catheter beyond the nasal introitus, and a CT scan that reveals <11 mm diameter of the pyriform aperture at the level of the inferior meatus. Initially, the airway is secured as in choanal atresia. Surgical correction occurs in the neonatal period via a sublabial approach to drill the pyriform aperture in order to widen it with the use of postoperative 3.5 mm ETT stents (Gnagi & Schraff 2013).

Oral cavity/oropharynx

As infants are obligate nasal breathers, oral cavity anomalies, such as cleft lip and palate, do not often result in neonatal airway distress. Micrognathia and retrognathia, particularly in the setting of severe Pierre Robin sequence (PRS), however, can result in respiratory distress. The following comprise PRS:

- Micrognathia
- Cleft palate
- Glossoptosis (**Figure 8.6**)

Pierre Robin sequence may occur as an isolated finding or may be part of a syndrome, most commonly the Stickler syndrome. In the neonatal period, PRS may result in respiratory distress and/or feeding difficulties. If the neonate is not in respiratory distress, management is typically conservative and consists of prone positioning with the possible adjuncts of a nasopharyngeal airway and/or a nasogastric tube. If the patient is in respiratory distress, after securing the airway,

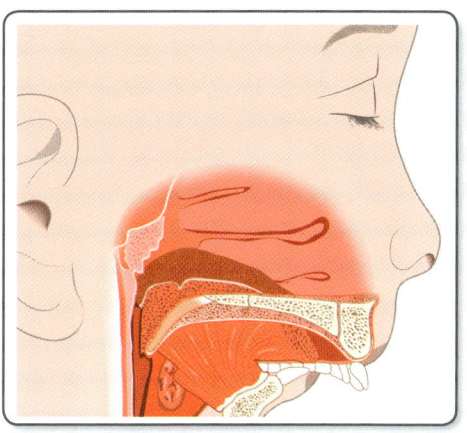

Figure 8.6 Drawing of airway obstruction created by the congenital anomalies associated with Pierre Robin Sequence.

management options include tongue–lip adhesion and mandibular distraction osteogenesis (Schaefer et al. 2004). In children with additional airway anomalies, neurologic, or pulmonary disease, a tracheostomy may prove necessary (**Figure 8.7**).

Larynx and trachea

Laryngomalacia

Laryngomalacia is the most common cause of infantile stridor, representing 45–75% of all congenital stridor (Landry & Thompson 2012). The male-to-female ratio is 2:1. The onset is within the first few weeks of life. Laryngomalacia peaks between 6 and 9 months and typically resolves by 12–24 months. The etiology is unknown, but the prevailing theory is neurologic, involving an immature or poorly integrated central nervous system during infancy. The patient presents with inspiratory stridor, which is worsened by agitation, supine positioning, and neck flexion. The patient often presents with concurrent feeding and vomiting symptoms. This is not surprising as 65–100% of laryngomalacia patients present with gastroesophageal reflux disease (GERD) (Landry & Thompson 2012). The diagnosis is made by history, physical examination, and flexible fiberoptic laryngoscopy (FFL). The FFL typically demonstrates some or all of the following findings: Ω-shaped epiglottis, redundant and prolapsing arytenoids, and foreshortened aryepiglottic folds (**Figure 8.8**). By performing FFL, other etiologies of inspiratory stridor, such as vocal fold paralysis or laryngeal cysts, may be ruled out. The management of laryngomalacia is three-tiered. If the patient is without feeding difficulties and has only mild laryngomalacia, they should simply be observed. If the patient has moderate laryngomalacia and feeding difficulties, they should typically receive acid suppression treatment and modification of feeds. If the patient has severe laryngomalacia that is unresponsive to medical management (approximately 10% of patients with laryngomalacia), they will require surgery. The most common surgery performed for

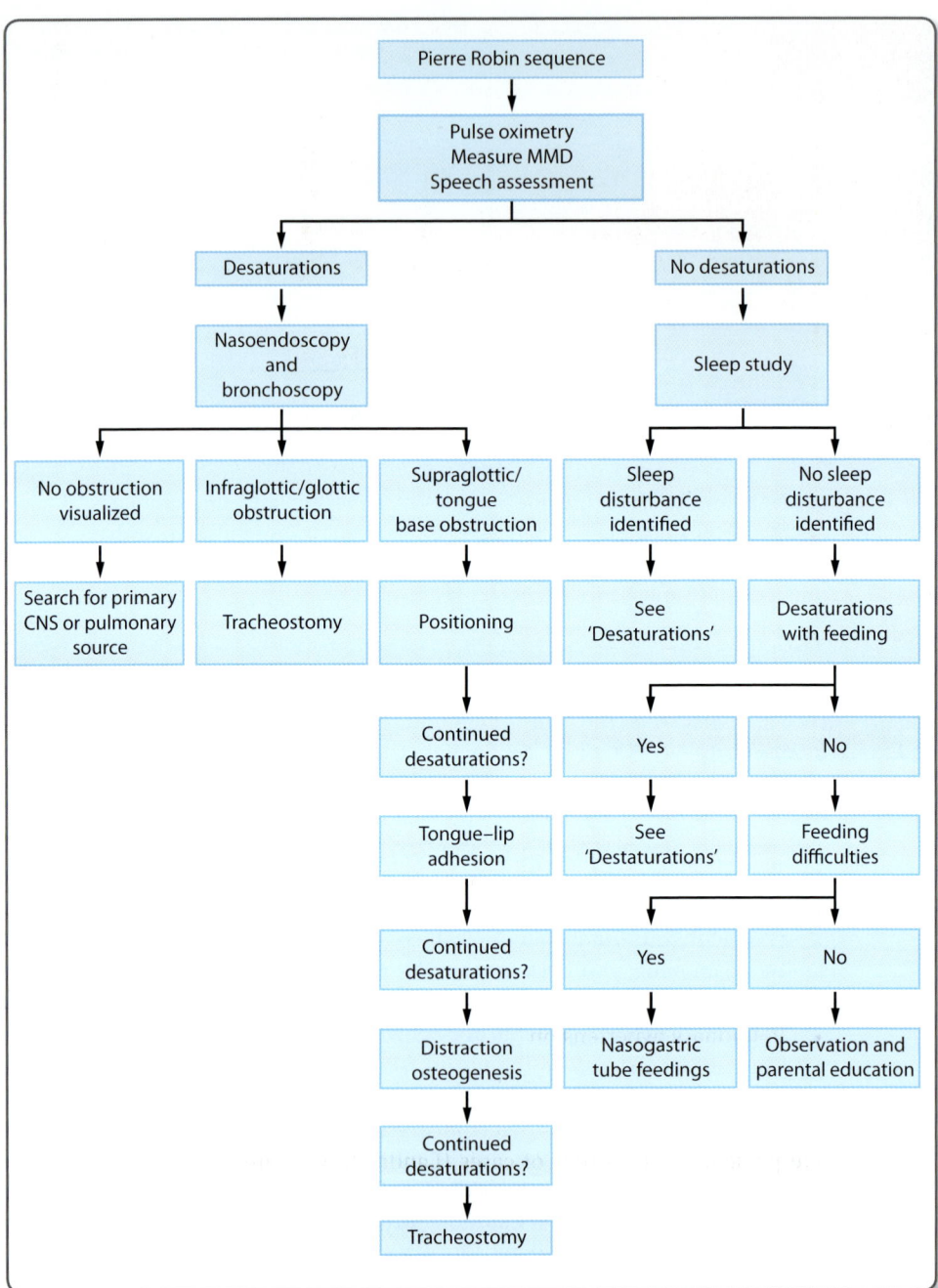

Figure 8.7 Algorithm for treating patients with isolated Pierre Robin sequence. MMD, maxillary-mandibular discrepancy; CNS, central nervous system. With permission from Schaefer RB, Stadler JA, Gosain AK. To distract or not to distract: an algorithm for airway management in isolated Pierre Robin Sequence. Plast Reconstr Surg 2004; 113:1113–1125.

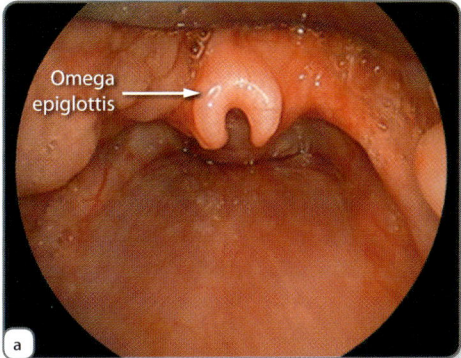

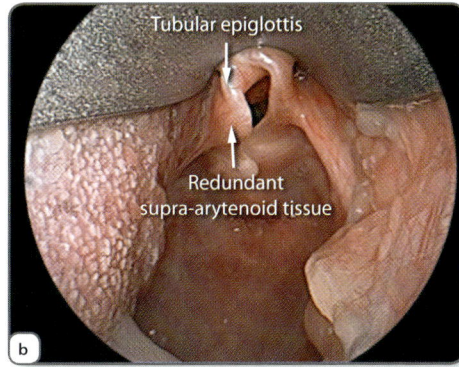

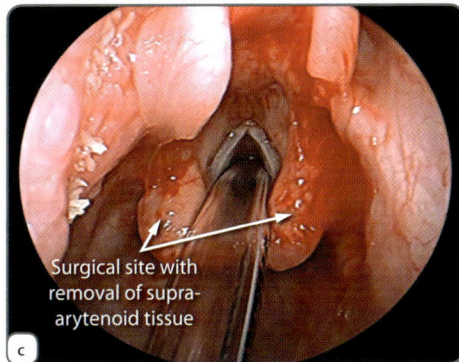

Figure 8.8 (a) An W-shaped epiglottis. (b) A tubular-shaped epiglottis along with redundant supra-arytenoid tissue, which is obstructing the glottis during inspiration. (c) The site of redundant supra-arytenoid tissue after surgical removal. With permission from Landry AM, Thompson DM. Laryngomalacia: disease presentation, spectrum, and management. Int J Ped 2012; 2012:753526. Epub 2012 Feb 27.

severe laryngomalacia is supraglottoplasty. The indications for surgery include severe stridor with any of the following:

- Failure to thrive
- Obstructive apnea
- Hypoxia
- Pectus excavatum
- Pulmonary hypertension
- Cor pulmonale

Prior to supraglottoplasty, direct laryngoscopy and bronchoscopy are performed to evaluate for secondary airway lesions, which are present in up to 64% of cases (Landry & Thompson 2012). The supraglottoplasty techniques involve microdissection and/or laser, and focus on correcting the site of collapse. Care must be taken to not overexcise mucosa, especially in the interarytenoid region, so as to avoid supraglottic scarring. Another major complication after supraglottoplasty is aspiration. Tracheostomy is reserved for patients in whom supraglottoplasty fails or for patients who have multiple comorbidities.

Bilateral vocal fold paralysis

In the newborn, bilateral vocal cord paralysis is fairly common for both vaginal and caesarian section deliveries. The etiology is thought to be an Erb's palsy type of traction injury on the recurrent nerve where it exits the skull base. In a series of 100 patients, recovery was seen in 90%, with persistence only in those with severe central neurological injury (Cohen et al. 1982). Patients present with a high-pitched crowing inspiratory stridor and respiratory distress. These children can be mask-ventilated easily, but intubation is usually necessary. During intubation, the cords can simply be pushed out of the way. If spontaneous resolution of the paralysis has occurred, tracheostomy frequently follows after 2 weeks. Typically, the tracheostomy tube is needed for 1–2 years. Regular re-evaluation is necessary because of the roughly 1–4% mortality from tracheostomy tubes. It is desirable to remove the tracheostomy tube as soon as the paralysis has resolved.

Laryngeal cysts

While laryngeal cysts are a rare cause of neonatal stridor, they must be considered in the differential diagnosis of stridor. The discussion of laryngeal cysts includes saccular cysts and ductal cysts. Symptoms of laryngeal cysts include stridor (70%), cough, cyanotic episodes, voice changes, and failure to thrive (Prowse & Knight 2012). While ductal cysts most commonly occur in the vallecula and are not anatomically part of the larynx, they are considered as laryngeal cysts because they often produce airway obstruction secondary to posterior displacement of the larynx (Prowse & Knight 2012) (**Figure 8.9**). Obstruction of the submucosal gland ducts produces ductal cysts, which comprise 75% of congenital airway cysts. Two thirds of vallecular cysts are associated with laryngomalacia (Prowse & Knight 2012). They often present with feeding difficulties and failure to thrive, and FFL provides the diagnosis.

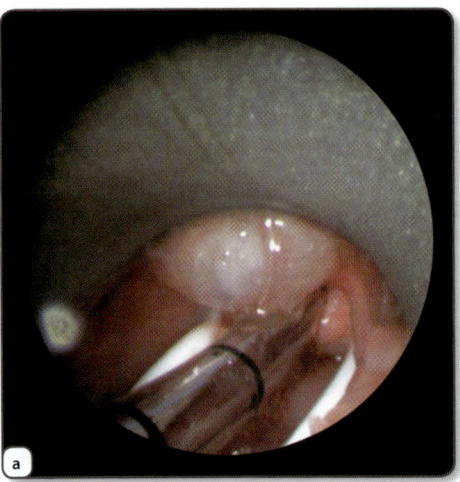 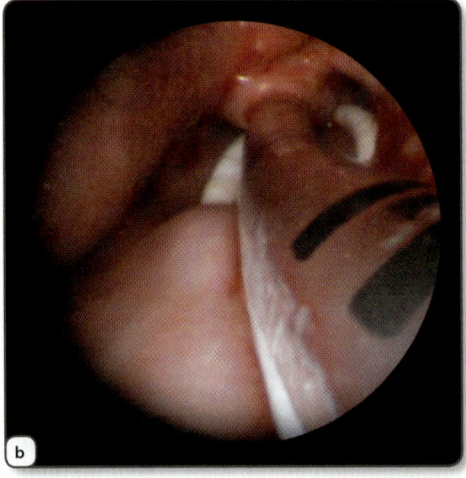

Figure 8.9 (a) Vallecular cyst prior to manipulation. (b) Vallecula after removal of the cyst by endoscopic marsupialization and carbon dioxide laser to the base of the cyst.

Treatment options include endoscopic excision, marsupialization, and laser ablation. Recurrence is fairly common, rendering surveillance necessary. Saccular cysts are less common than ductal cysts and present earlier with more severe airway compromise. Saccular cysts are described as dilated, mucus-filled saccules of the laryngeal ventricle. Lateral saccular cysts are most common and may extend laterally via the thyrohyoid membrane into the neck. Diagnosis involves FFL and direct laryngoscopy. Treatment may occur via endoscopic marsupialization, laser excision, or transcervical approaches for large or recurrent saccular cysts. Postoperative observation is important, as recurrence is known to occur.

Hemangiomas

Hemangiomas are the most common pediatric head and neck neoplasm, but constitute only 1% of congenital laryngeal neoplasms. The natural course of hemangiomas is a rapid proliferation stage over the first year of life followed by an involution stage over the next 10–12 years (Ida et al. 2008). Women are twice as likely to be afflicted as men. The etiology is thought to involve mesodermal rests of vasoformative tissue. Patients often present in the first 8 weeks to 6 months of life with biphasic stridor, intermittent respiratory distress, croup-like coughing, and feeding difficulties. Of patients with airway hemangiomas, 50% have other cutaneous hemangiomas. Diagnosis is made by history, physical examination, direct laryngoscopy, and bronchoscopy. The hemangioma most often appears as a unilateral, single sessile, compressible, bluish-pink mass in the subglottis (**Figure 8.10**). After diagnosis, some advocate for an MRI to detect extralaryngeal and intracranial hemangiomas (Javia et al. 2011). As spontaneous regression is possible, observation may be possible for very small hemangiomas, but careful observation is necessary. There are a variety of medical, endoscopic, and open techniques available to manage laryngeal hemangiomas. Propranolol, a nonselective β-2 antagonist,

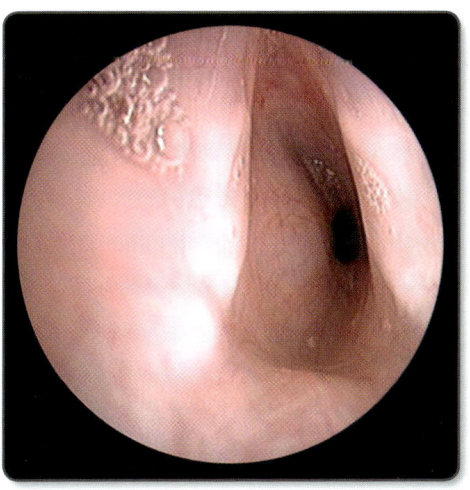

Figure 8.10 Endoscopic view showing a unilateral, smooth swelling in the subglottis, the classical appearance of a subglottic hemangioma. With permission from Bajaj Y, Kapoor K, Ifeacho S, et al. Great Ormond Street Hospital treatment guidelines for use of propranolol in infantile isolated subglottic haemangioma. J Laryngol Otol 2013; 127:295–298.

has demonstrated efficacy in producing hemangioma regression. There are cardiovascular risks associated with its use, of which hypotension, bradycardia, and hypoglycemia are the most prominent ones (Bajaj et al. 2013). Electrocardiogram and echocardiogram, as well as an extensive history and physical examination, are performed prior to its use. Propranolol is often used over a course of 12 months, with serial endoscopic evaluations used to assess hemangioma regression. The Great Ormond Street Hospital in London has published its protocol (**Figure 8.11**). Other treatment modalities include steroids (systemic or intralesional), laser endoscopic ablation, open resection, and, in severe cases, tracheostomy with observation. Long-term follow-up of hemagioma patients is advocated.

Stenosis

Congenital laryngotracheal stenosis (LTS) is a less common cause of neonatal stridor. The majority of LTS is acquired from etiologies, such as intubation trauma, caustic ingestion, and GERD. Failure of the recanalization process during fetal airway embryogenesis is thought to produce congenital airway stenosis (**Figure 8.12**). Complete atresia may occur and requires management with an ex utero intrapartum treatment (EXIT) procedure. Congenital LTS is often associated with syndromes such as 22q11 deletion, CHARGE, trisomy 21, and Fraser (Blanchard et al. 2013). Patients with LTS present with stridor within the first few weeks of life, a croup-like cough, and hoarse cry. If the stenosis is severe, then the patient may present with respiratory distress. Diagnosis is made by endoscopic evaluation of the laryngotracheal tree. Subglottic stenosis is defined by a subglottic diameter <4 mm in a

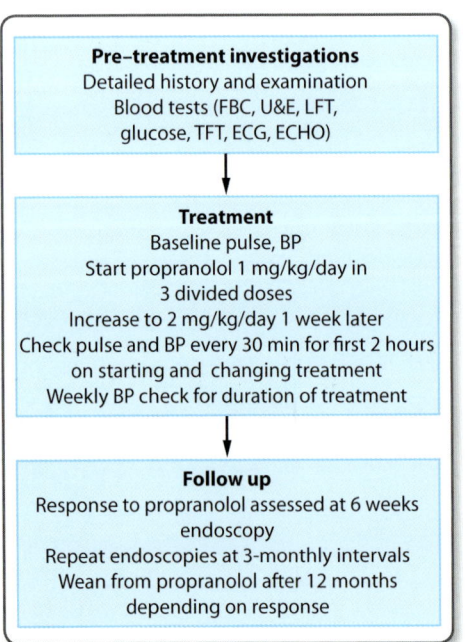

Pre–treatment investigations
Detailed history and examination
Blood tests (FBC, U&E, LFT,
glucose, TFT, ECG, ECHO)

↓

Treatment
Baseline pulse, BP
Start propranolol 1 mg/kg/day in
3 divided doses
Increase to 2 mg/kg/day 1 week later
Check pulse and BP every 30 min for first 2 hours
on starting and changing treatment
Weekly BP check for duration of treatment

↓

Follow up
Response to propranolol assessed at 6 weeks
endoscopy
Repeat endoscopies at 3-monthly intervals
Wean from propranolol after 12 months
depending on response

Figure 8.11 Flow chart for propranolol treatment for infantile subglottic hemangioma. FBC, full blood count; U&E, urea and electrolyte analysis; LFT, liver function tests; TFT, thyroid function tests; ECG, electrocardiography; ECHO, echocardiography; BP, blood pressure. With permission from Bajaj Y, Kapoor K, Ifeacho S, et al. Great Ormond Street Hospital treatment guidelines for use of propranolol in infantile isolated subglottic haemangioma. J Laryngol Otol 2013; 127:295–298.

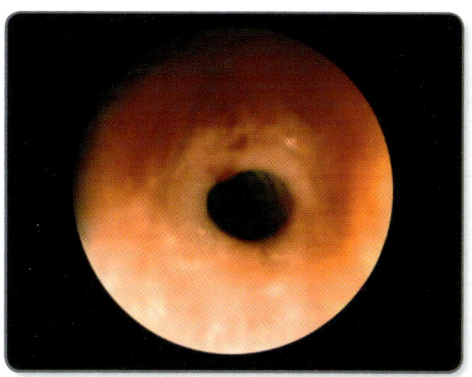

Figure 8.12 Cartilaginous congenital subglottic stenosis. The cricoid ring is regularly shaped, but small. Note the normal-sized tracheal rings distal to the cricoid cartilage. Ida JB, Guarisco JL, Rodriguez KH, Amedee RG. Obstructive lesions of the pediatric subglottis. Ochsner J 2008; 8:119–128.

term infant and <3 mm in a premature infant. The Myer–Cotton grading system classifies the severity of the stenosis based on the degree of obstruction, with Grade I being mild, Grade II being moderate, Grade III being severe, and Grade IV being no detectable lumen (**Table 8.1**). Secondary airway lesions are also sought during endoscopy. If the patient is in respiratory distress and has severe laryngeal or subglottic stenosis unresponsive to endoscopic management, an emergency tracheostomy may be necessary to stabilize the airway. Management involves observation with Grade I to mild Grade II stenosis. If GERD is thought to be present, aggressive acid suppression therapy is started. For moderate Grade II to Grade III stenosis, endoscopic techniques involving laser or cold steel division of the stenosis and balloon dilation are often advocated as initial procedures. Each of the endoscopic techniques may be used separately, but often balloon dilation follows either laser or cold steel division (**Figure 8.13**). Steroid injection and mitomycin C, an inhibitory alkylating agent, are adjuvants that may also be used in conjunction with the endoscopic techniques (Sinacori et al. 2013). Recurrence often occurs, and repeated endoscopic procedures may prove necessary. Anterior cricoid split is an alternative option in premature infants and in neonates. More definitive management of refractory and severe LTS occurs with the open technique of laryngotracheal reconstruction. Laryngotracheal reconstruction may involve single and double stages, anterior and posterior grafts, and the use of stents. Decannulation rates tend to be high after open repair.

Table 8.1 Myer–Cotton grading scale for subglottic stenosis	
Grade	Obstruction (%)
I	<50
II	51–70
III	71–99
IV	100

From Ida JB, Guarisco JL, Rodriguez KH, Amedee RG. Obstructive lesions of the pediatric subglottis. Ochsner J 2008; 8:119–128.

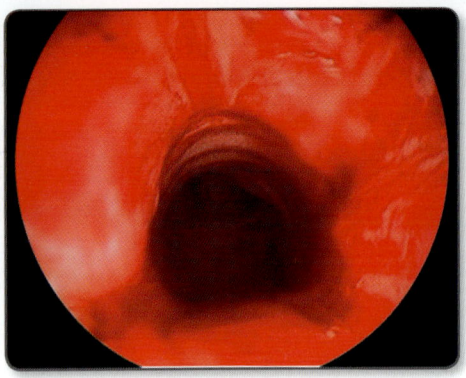

Figure 8.13 Subglottic stenosis after carbon dioxide laser incision as well as balloon dilation. With permission from Sinacori JR, Taliercio SJ, Duong E, Benson C. Modalities of treatment for laryngotracheal stenosis: the EVMS experience. Laryngoscope 2013; 123:3131–3136.

Conclusion

Pediatric airway management relies on knowledge of the key anatomic and physiologic differences present in infants and children. Specialized instrumentation and equipment allow improved assessment and management of the pediatric airway. Congenital anomalies affect every level of the airway. Thorough knowledge of the natural history, signs/symptoms, diagnosis, and management of congenital airway abnormalities is required for its safe and effective treatment.

References

American Heart Association. Part 12: pediatric advanced life support. Circulation 2005; 112:IV-167-IV-187.

Bajaj Y, Kapoor K, Ifeacho S, et al. Great Ormond Street Hospital treatment guidelines for use of propranolol in infantile isolated subglottic haemangioma. J Laryngol Otol 2013; 127:295–298.

Blanchard M, Leboulanger N, Thierry B, et al. Management specificities of congenital laryngeal stenosis: external and endoscopic approaches. Laryngoscope 2014; 124: 1013–1018.

Bluestone CD, Stool SE, Alper CM, et al. Pediatric otolaryngology, 4th edn. Philadelphia, PA: Saunders, 2003:1366–1370.

Cote CJ, Lerman J, Anderson BJ. A practice of anesthesia for infants and children, 5th edn. Philadelphia, PA: Saunders; 2013:237–276.

Cohen SR, Geller KA, Birns JW, Thompson JW. Laryngeal paralysis in children: a long-term retrospective study. Ann Otol Rhinol Laryngol 1982; 91:417–424.

Gnagi SH, Schraff SA. Nasal obstruction in newborns. Ped Clin N Am 2013; 60:903–922.

Ida JB, Guarisco JL, Rodriguez KH, Amedee RG. Obstructive lesions of the pediatric subglottis. Ochsner J 2008; 8:119–128.

Javia LR, Zur KB, Jacobs IN. Evolving treatments in the management of laryngotracheal hemangiomas: will propranolol supplant steroids and surgery? Int J Pediatr Otorhinolaryngol 2011; 75:1450–1454.

Landry AM, Thompson DM. Laryngomalacia: disease presentation, spectrum, and management. Int J Pediatr 2012; 2012:753526, 6 pages.

Prowse S, Knight L. Congenital cysts of the infant larynx. Int J Pediatr Otorhinolaryngol 2012; 76:708–711.

Schaefer RB, Stadler JA, Gosain AK. To distract or not to distract: an algorithm for airway management in isolated Pierre Robin Sequence. Plast Reconstr Surg 2004; 113:1113–1125.

Sinacori JR, Taliercio SJ, Duong E, Benson C. Modalities of treatment for laryngotracheal stenosis: the EVMS experience. Laryngoscope 2013; 123:3131–3136.

Further reading

Bluestone CD, Rosenfeld RM. Surgical atlas of pediatric otolaryngology. Hamilton: BC Decker Inc, 2002.

<table>
<tr><td>9</td><td>

Pediatric airway management part 2: management of airway emergencies

</td></tr>
</table>

Jerome W Thompson, Rose Mary Stocks, Jennifer McLevy

Airway foreign bodies

Airway foreign bodies are by far the most deadly and difficult airway situation to manage. To deal with these obstructions, one must break the airway down into four segments in order to localize the obstruction: (i) nasal, (ii) oropharyngeal, (iii) laryngeal, and (iv) tracheobronchial. Nasal foreign bodies in children are very common and are usually plastic, foam or vegetable matter. Their danger comes only from subsequent sepsis or dislodgement into the lower airway. Hartmann packing forceps are ideal for removal of these objects (**Figure 9.1**).

Oropharyngeal foreign bodies are far more dangerous, produce immediate obstruction, and may require an emergent tracheotomy to get below the obstruction (**Figure 9.2**). In children, these are usually the result of a bizarre accident or foul play.

Laryngeal foreign bodies are either acutely partially or totally obstructive; seldom are they chronic (**Figures 9.3** and **9.4**). All must be cared for in the operating room via direct rigid laryngoscopy with stout forceps that are able to remove the foreign body immediately. Broken glass, seed husks, and plastic fingernails have become wedged between the vocal cords and removed safely. Larger nonflat foreign

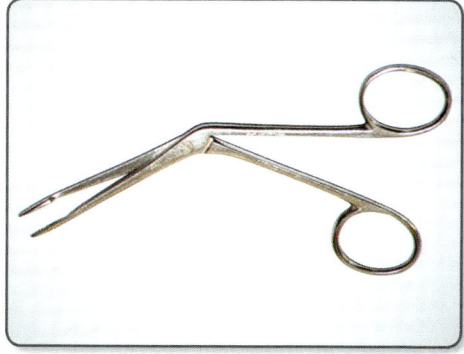

Figure 9.1 Hartmann packing forceps for nasal foreign bodies.

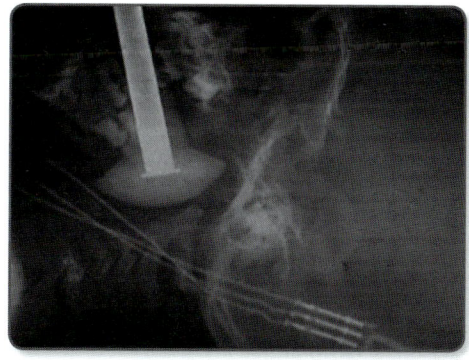

Figure 9.2 Fatal baton in pharynx.

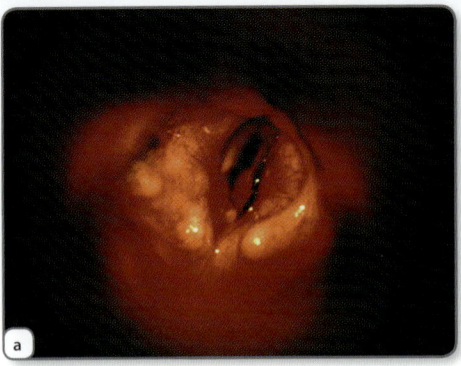
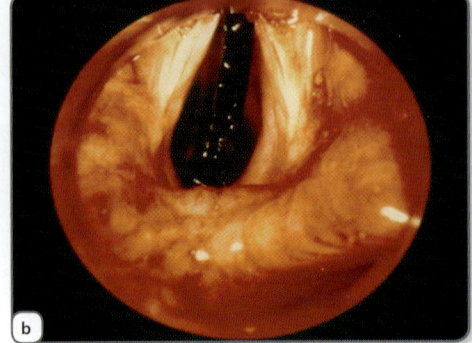

Figure 9.3 (a and b) Glass foreign body in the larynx.

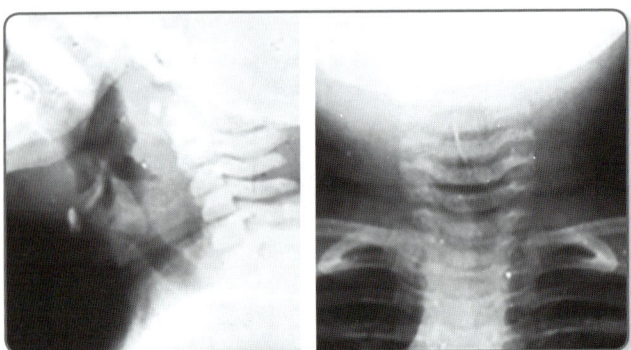

Figure 9.4 Glass foreign body on lateral X-ray in larynx.

bodies coughed up from below in the trachea and impacted into the funnel-shaped subglottis are frequently fatal. This is because the vocal cords are not the narrowest part of the airway, but rather it is the conus elasticus of the subglottis that is the most restrictive area (this is the conical junction between the trachea and the cricoid cartilage of the larynx). Dealing with tracheobronchial foreign bodies (TFBs) requires a great deal of skill and speed. The status of the patient must be accurately assessed, instruments prepared, and proper anesthesia administered. Remember that a spontaneous breathing patient is safer than an apneic one. A rigid laryngoscope and bronchoscope are used for airway foreign body removal. Frequently, the object may move around within the trachea and into either bronchus (usually the right), depending on its size. If large, it may form a 'ball valve' within the trachea and periodically completely obstruct it. If it is too big to remove through the cords, it must be removed via emergent tracheotomy. Seeds and popcorn kernels can swell with tracheobronchial moisture to several times their original size and become lodged in this manner. If the object is smaller, but still blocking the trachea, it can be forced into one of the two bronchi, allowing ventilation of at least one lung (**Figure**

9.5). Once the position of the foreign body is stable in the bronchi, the patient can be paralyzed and the object can be crushed into smaller fragments and removed. Most operating rooms have an impressive array of bronchoscopic tools for crushing, biting, and removal of TFBs (**Figure 9.6**). Nuts, once crushed, release oils that are highly inflammatory and will produce a temporary white-out of the effected lung. It is prudent to lavage out the entire detectable fragment once the TFB is crushed and removed (Zur & Litman 2009). Occasionally, the TFB will have to be rotated or repositioned to align the tapered aspect so that it will pass through the subglottis and cords. If it is made of a hard material that cannot be crushed, the practitioner should first try to pull it through the cords; if that fails, then emergent adequate tracheotomy is needed. Rarely is a thoracotomy necessary.

Trauma

Nasal and midface

Nasal and midface trauma are common in children, and usually do not encroach on the airway. Those who are nasally intubating need to be aware of the risk of intracranial passage of the endotracheal tube if the cribriform plate or skull base is fractured (**Figure 9.7**). Direct visualization with a fiberoptic nasopharyngoscope with an endotracheal tube over it is a good alternative to blind passage of the tube (**Figure 9.8**). Perhaps, the most challenging aspect of intubation in these cases is the management of the associated hemorrhage. Two soft inflatable epistaxis catheters passed into the floor of the nose, into the nasopharynx, and then inflated, will often stem the flow of blood into the oropharynx (**Figure 9.9**). They form a posterior nasal pack and can

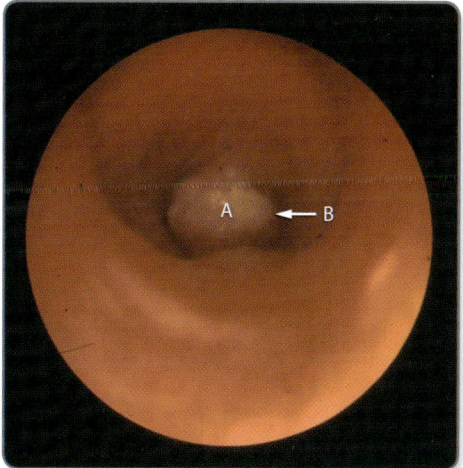

Figure 9.5 (A) Tracheal foreign body. (B) Bronchial foreign body pushed into right mainstem.

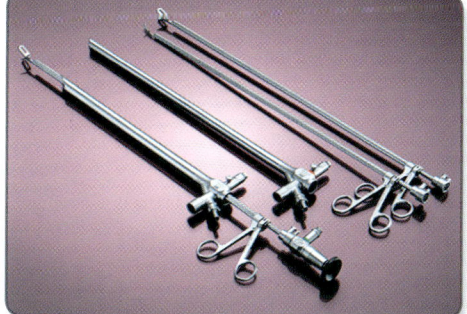

Figure 9.6 Assorted bronchoscopy instruments. (©2014 Photo by courtesy of Karl Storz Endoscopy-America, Inc.)

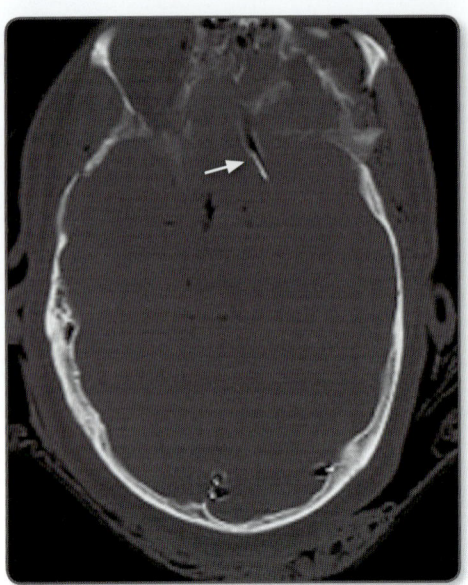

Figure 9.7 Nasogastric tube (arrow) in the brain through the cribriform plate.

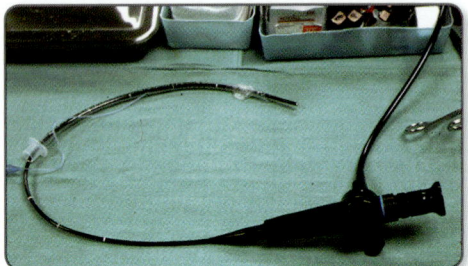

Figure 9.8 Nasopharyngoscope with endotracheal tube slide over outside for flexible fiberoptic intubation.

cause bradycardia by stimulating baroreceptors in the nasopharynx (Rashid & Karagama 2010). Control can be difficult, but the airway can be visualized with adequate suction and the patient orally intubated.

Soft palate

Punctures to the soft palate are less of an airway problem than a vascular one. A rule of thumb is that if the puncture is lateral to the anterior tonsillar pillar's edge, then a carotid angiogram should be performed (**Figure 9.10**). Otherwise, the puncture should be explored for retained fragments, closed, and the patient prescribed a course of antibiotics.

Jaw

Mandible fractures produce airway obstruction in several ways. First, there can be significant hemorrhage into the airway that must be

Figure 9.9 Nasopharyngeal epistaxis catheter (by courtesy of Atos Medical AB Sweden).

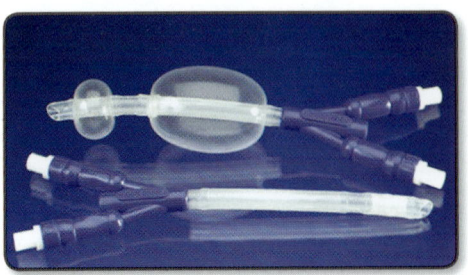

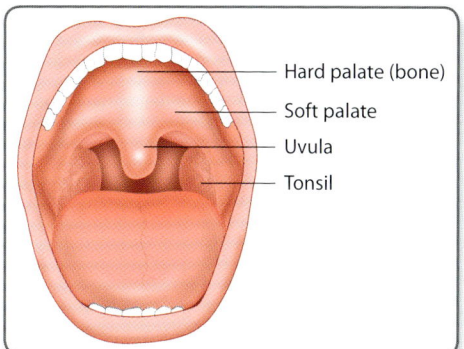

Figure 9.10 Palate puncture line of demarcation (see text).

Hard palate (bone)

Soft palate

Uvula

Tonsil

managed, occasionally via tracheotomy. Hemorrhage is usually due to the inferior alveolar artery being disrupted. Second, tongue swelling can obstruct the airway. Third, trismus limits opening the mouth and restricts access to the airway. A broken jaw can be easily moved out of the way for intubation under general anesthesia. The fracture site can act like another 'hinge' to open the airway. Once the fracture is reapproximated, either temporarily or permanently with plates and screws, bleeding usually subsides.

Larynx

Laryngeal trauma is extremely dangerous because there is usually airway obstruction, if not immediately, then later from swelling and edema. There are five groups of laryngeal trauma correlating the degree of injury and the extent of surgical intervention (**Table 9.1**). Commonly, there is free air in the neck if there is a mucosal tear (**Figure 9.11**). This is a good indicator that there has been significant structural injury, and a close examination with a rigid laryngoscopy is indicated. Injuries can include minor mucosal tears, arytenoid dislocation, vocal cord avulsion, structural thyroid and cricoid cartilage fractures, displacement or a combination of some or all of these. The first treatment should be to secure the airway with a tracheotomy, and then to explore the larynx through a horizontal incision. Keep in mind that vascular injuries can also occur and an arteriogram should be obtained

Table 9.1 Laryngeal trauma classification system	
Group	**Characteristics**
1	Minor endolaryngeal hematomas or lacerations in absence of detectable fracture.
2	Edema, hematoma, minor mucosal disruption without exposed cartilage, varying degrees of airway compromise; nondisplaced fracture(s).
3	Massive edema, large mucosal lacerations, exposed cartilage, vocal cord immobility, displaced fractures.
4	As group 3 but greater severity, with disruption of anterior larynx, unstable fractures, ≥2 fracture lines, severe mucosal injuries.
5	Complete laryngotracheal separation.

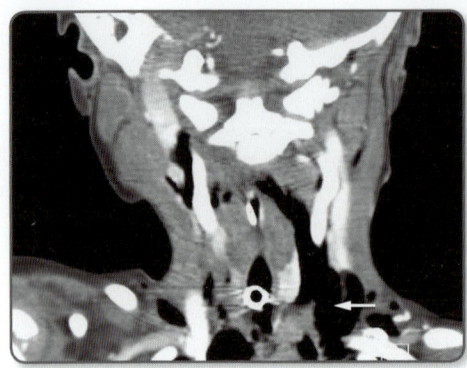

Figure 9.11 Free air in the neck (arrow) from laryngotracheal puncture.

as soon as practicable once the patient's airway is secure. Arytenoid dislocations must be repositioned and they may still produce a poor voice outcome (Stack & Ridley 1994). For more severe injuries to the larynx, a midline laryngofissure approach is necessary (**Figure 9.12**). Avulsed vocal cords should be reapproximated to their original insertion on the thyroid lamina and stented. Mucosal tears should be repaired with absorbable sutures, and cartilage framework fractures should be stabilized either with permanent sutures or with miniplates and be stented. The screws in these plates will loosen in the cartilage and may need to be removed, with the plates, in 3–6 months (**Figure 9.13**). Stenting is almost always necessary for up to 2 weeks.

Trachea

Tracheal tears may occur from blunt force to the neck or chest or even by a balloon used to dilate the airway. Usually, the tear is along the

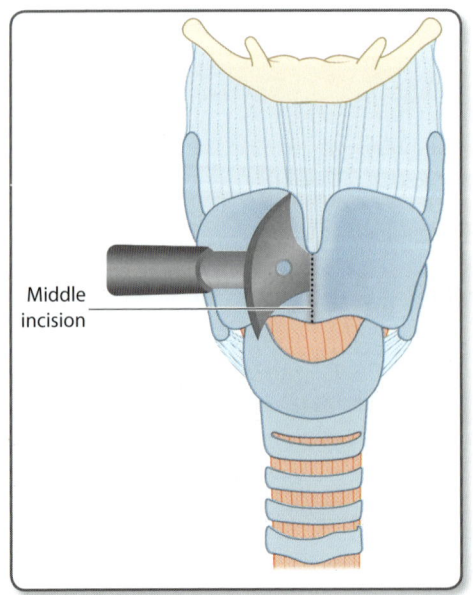

Middle incision

Figure 9.12 Laryngofissure for access to the vocal cords.

weaker posterior tracheal wall and is linear (**Figure 9.14**). If the patient is stable, on low vent settings, and has chest tubes in place to manage the escaping air, the tear will seal in 72 hours and heal completely within a week with good antibiotic coverage. Neck exploration or thoracotomy is frequently not necessary, but if performed, then primary closure with a muscle flap to seal the tear and make it airtight is required. Bronchial tears from balloon dilation have also been observed and successfully treated conservatively. It is not uncommon to have post-traumatic air in the neck and chest after a high-speed blunt trauma without an obvious tear on endoscopy (Ladurner et al. 2005). These, after close endoscopic inspection for esophageal involvement, can be managed conservatively. The mechanism of this extravasation air is thought to be a sudden high-pressure blast of air from neck or chest compression pushing though a micro air dissection path along a tracheal or bronchial vessel in the cartilaginous or muscular wall, and then connecting into the pleural or neck space. Sometimes, the amount of air in the chest is so small that a chest tube is not necessary. These patients usually do well. Even moderate amounts of air can be observed and well resolved.

Laryngotracheal separation or clothesline injuries are fairly common in areas where open motorized sports vehicle-based and cross-country activities occur (**Figure 9.15**). The mechanism is that an individual moving at high speed with no protection for the anterior neck encounters a low-hanging rope or wire that strikes them across the neck in a very narrow band at the level of the trachea. The mechanism of separation is that the trachea is pinned against the vertebral column and separates because the lower trachea is tethered by intrathoracic structures and cannot 'give'. Patients who make it to the hospital have stridor, free air in the neck, with a telltale horizontal ecchymosis across the anterior

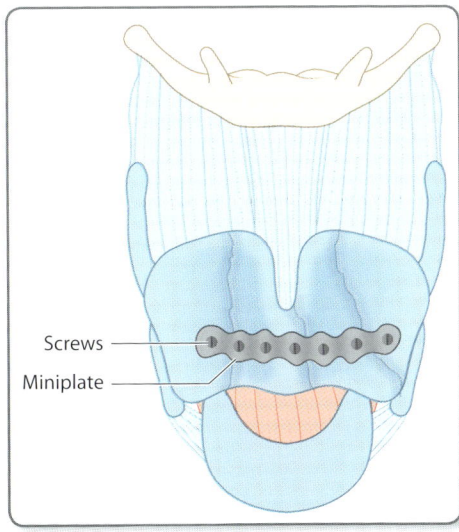

Screws
Miniplate

Figure 9.13 Plating of thyroid cartilage.

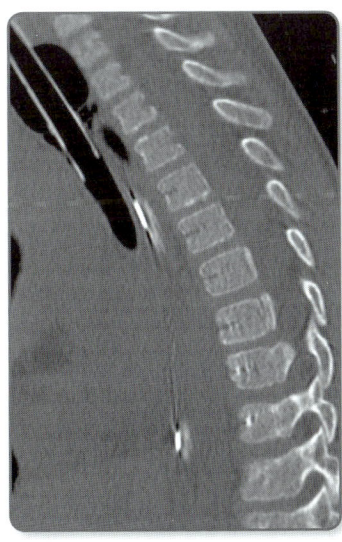

Figure 9.14 Posterior tracheal wall tear.

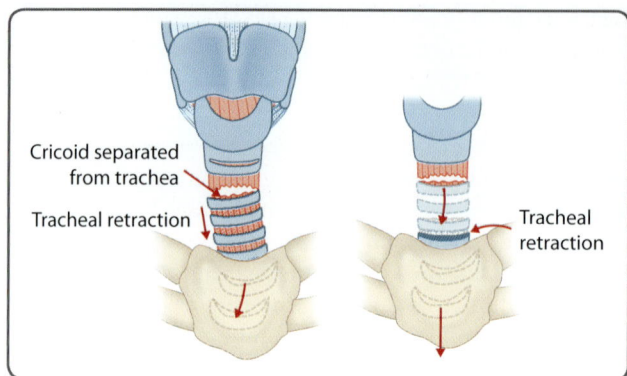

Figure 9.15 Tracheal separation.

neck. Some are amazingly asymptomatic. Emergent rigid bronchoscopy is necessary, as are chest tubes. The bronchoscope must not be passed beyond the separation into the distal segment. It needs to be held steady at the separation site to demarcate the upper section and to provide ventilation to the patient while the neck is opened in an emergent fashion for tracheostomy. Because of the nature of the separation, there may have been retraction of the distal segment into a retrosternal position, so the tracheotomy incision should be low, just above the sternal notch. The dissection goes down the midline and follows the air bubbles. Once the distal end has been located, it is secured to the skin, an endotracheal tube is passed, and the patient is then paralyzed. With the patient stable, other appropriate diagnostic procedures can be performed to evaluate for vascular injury. Reanastomosis of the separated ends of the trachea can then be considered. A fiberoptic laryngoscopy is performed since the recurrent nerves are usually severed as well. An extended neck flap incision is made and the neck explored. Frequently, a hyoid release is necessary to relieve the tension on the closure. Primary end-to-end anastomosis usually results in some degree of circumferential stenosis, so a spatulated repair is suggested if possible, with slow absorbing sutures. If Prolene is used and accidently enters the lumen, it can cause prolonged granulation tissue.

Neck

Slash lacerations to neck are common. If stable, the arteriogram is crucial to rule out carotid or jugular injury. Not infrequently, the trachea is open and can be intubated through the laceration and repaired later. If the airway is secure and bleeding is controlled, then an arteriogram should be performed first, followed by exploration. If there is no time to do this and the great vessels are obviously injured, immediate surgery is necessary with the understanding that vascular surgery support needs to be available for reconstruction after the hemorrhage had been controlled. Many structures may have been injured, including the larynx, trachea, vessels, muscles, and nerves. Computed tomography (CT) is critical (Shafer & Brown 1983). Each specific structure needs to be sought out and repaired (**Figure 9.16**).

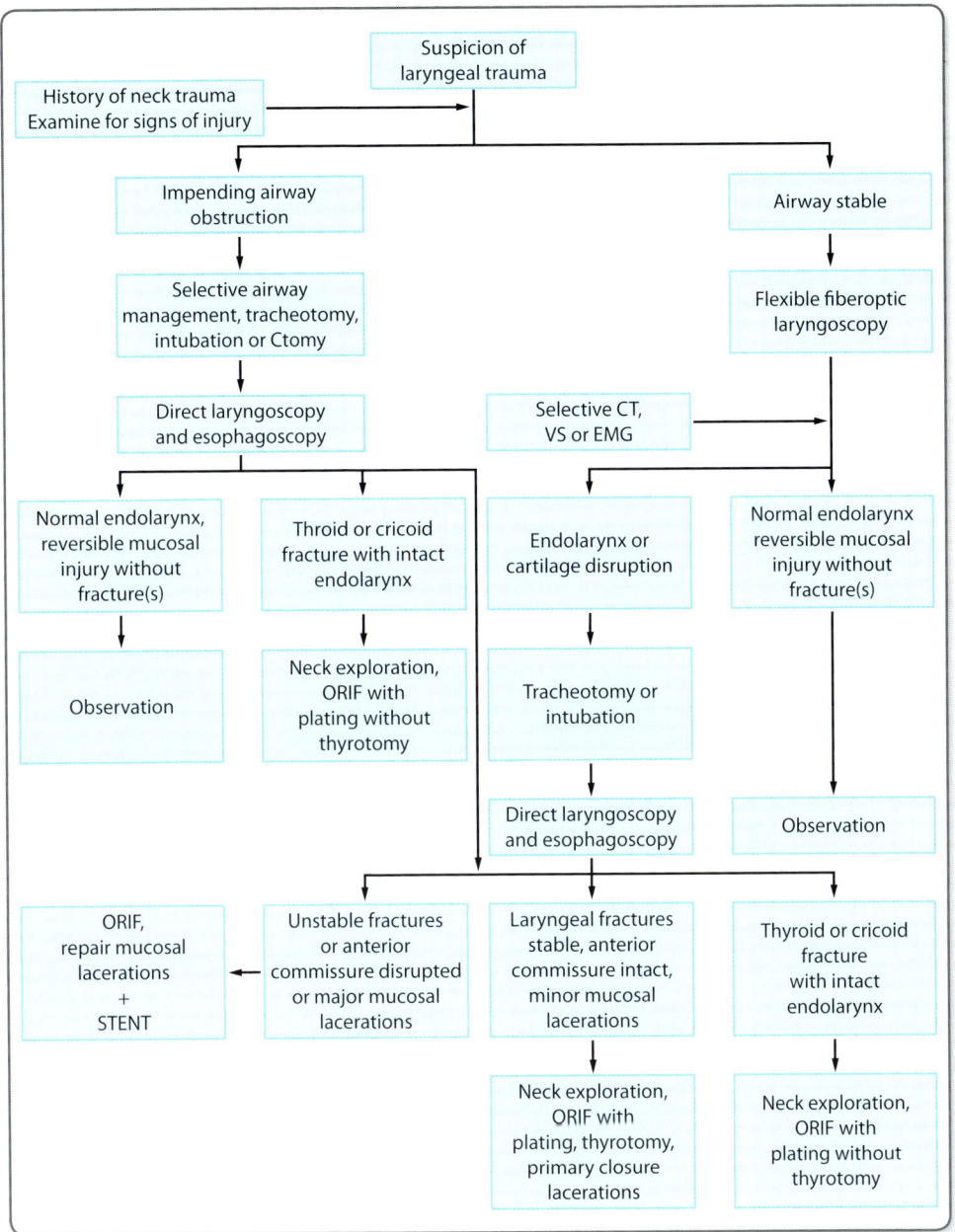

Figure 9.16 Neck exploration protocol. CT, computed tomography; Ctomy, cricothyrotomy; EMG, electromyography of the larynx; ORIF, open reduction and internal fixation of laryngeal skeletal fractures; STENT, endolaryngeal stent or lumen keeper; VS, videostroboscopy of larynx.

Burns to face, neck and airway

Burns to the airway gained the most recognition after two events in the 1940s: the Cocoanut Grove fire and soldiers injured in World War II. Most of the injuries and deaths from the fire were inhalational as were the soldiers' (Robinson & Miller 1986). There are three major components responsible for injury to the airway. The first is chemical, from the aldehydes, ammonia, and hydrochloric acid vapors in smoke. The second is from the direct thermal injury denaturing proteins. The third is potentially most dangerous: the infectious process that always follows an airway burn. Smoke temperatures range from 260°C to 280°C, but anything about 150°C will injure mucous membrane. Usually, the upper airway structures incur the most severe burns, while it is less common for the trachea and lungs to be injured. In severe circumstances, though, the entire airway is involved. Aggressive pulmonary toilet for the pulmonary thermal injury is necessary via an endotracheal tube. Tracheotomy is usually avoided or delayed because of the secondary infection of the adjacent neck skin and subsequent sepsis. Frequent bronchoscopies to remove carbonaceous material are also necessary. Long-term sequelae include a permanent disruption of the mucosal transport system. The damage to the airway is usually due to the prolonged intubation and rarely to the burn itself. However, scarring and stenosis of the true vocal cords, subglottis, and trachea can result in obstruction of the airway and may require later reconstruction.

Caustic ingestion

Caustic ingestions should be treated in the same way as inhalational burns, with the added concern about damage to the esophagus and stomach. The caustic agent can acutely cause severe tongue, pharyngeal, and epiglottic swelling, as well as laryngeal injury and obstruction. Intubation at the least and possibly tracheotomy are necessary if endoscopy shows severe burns through the mucosa into the cartilage or muscle. The use of steroids and antibiotics is controversial, but is usually helpful in most cases.

Infection

Ludwig's angina

Ludwig's angina is a sudden and potentially fatal illness, described nearly 200 years ago by Wilhelm Friedrich von Ludwig in 1836 (Busch & Shah 1997). It has been known by several other names: angina Ludovici, angina Maligna, and morbus Strangularia. The word 'angina' comes from the Greek word 'ankhon' that means strangling, thus 'Ludwig's strangling illness'. The mechanism is sudden swelling or cellulitis of the tissues in the floor of mouth and adjacent anterior neck. There is a diffuse accumulation of interstitial fluid in these structures and in the fascial spaces on either side of the mylohyoid muscle, which acts as an impenetrable barrier. This migration of fluid into the sublingual and submandibular space dramatically increases the functional volume of these areas, thus thrusting the overlaying tongue superiorly, and occasional out of the mouth altogether (**Figure 9.17**). In addition, because the tongue muscles are attached to the hyoid bone, the hydraulic expansion also rotates the tongue posteriorly, occluding the oropharynx and closing the upper airway, producing the sensation of strangulation and eventually actual suffocation. The interstitial fluid can be best seen on a CT scan, where the tissues have a characteristic 'stranding' or filamentous appearance holding them together with fluid in between (**Figure 9.18**). The tongue is elevated against the hard and soft palate and occasionally completely against the posterior oropharyngeal wall, which is buttressed by the vertebral bodies. No abscess cavity is seen on imaging or ultrasound. The infection is caused by bacterial organisms, usually streptococcal or staphylococcal species, but other bacteria such as the gram-negative organisms (*Neisseria catarrhalis, Escherichia coli, Pseudomonas aeruginosa,* and *Haemophilus influenzae)* and anaerobic bacteria such as peptostreptococci or *Fusobacterium nucleatum* can also cause this infection. Piercing of the frenulum and tongue has recently been associated with Ludwig's angina. The first symptom is fever as the manifestation of a bacterial infection of diffuse discomfort in the anterior neck and with tongue movement and progressively more severe pain, followed by the physical findings of swelling of the upper anterior neck (submental triangle) or 'bull neck'. Swallowing becomes difficult (dysphagia), and saliva accumulates in the oral cavity. Severe malaise results and, in severe late or untreated cases, difficulty breathing, with audible obstructed airway sounds (stridor) both to and fro with the decreasing air movement. Early treatment is medical, with aggressive intravenous high dose antibiotics with combined gram-negative anaerobe and gram-positive coverage. Should the airway become compromised, the American Society of Anesthesiologist Difficult Airway Algorithm should be followed, using fiberoptic or GlideScope intubation. If these should fail, or prolonged

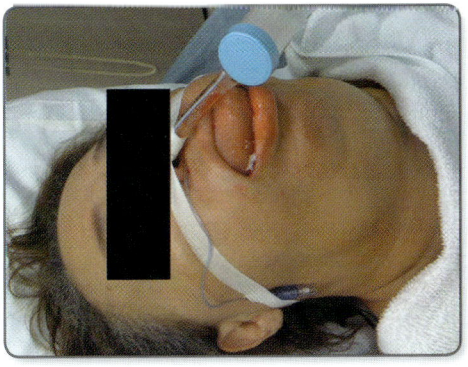

Figure 9.17 Ludwig's angina tongue.

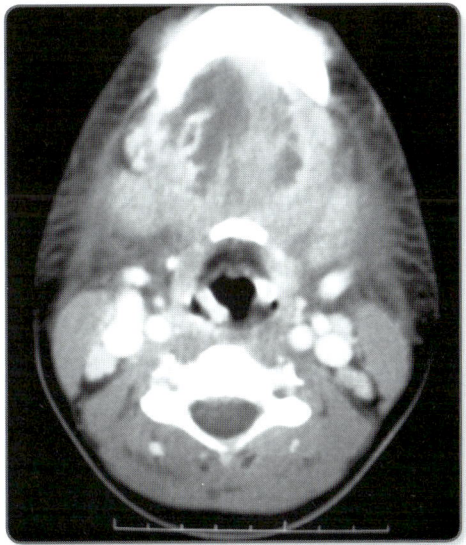

Figure 9.18 X-ray of Ludwig's angina.

airway support is not possible in the facility, then a tracheotomy should be performed. Surgical drainage of the submental triangle is achieved with a drain placed through the mylohyoid muscle. Very little fluid will be found initially, but more will drain slowing out over the ensuing days. Recovery should be complete within a week.

Epiglottitis

Epiglottitis is a disease traditionally caused by *Haemophilus influenzae B* in children and was common until vaccination almost completely eliminated it in developed countries. Now, other pathogens such as highly resistant *Staphylococcus aureus* are far more prevalent, especially in immunocompromised patients. The condition presents in a classic fashion with sudden onset high fever, hoarseness, inspiratory stridor, and drooling due to an inability to swallow (**Figure 9.19**). The patient may present leaning forward in order to breathe more freely, in the classic 'tripod' position. In the past century, tracheotomy was the treatment of choice, but with advanced intubation techniques and equipment, intubation is now the first choice, followed by tracheotomy if that fails.

Tracheitis

Tracheitis is a bacterial infection that produces a thick inflammatory exudate along the entire tracheal wall. The exudate sloughs off and obstructs the tracheal lumen. The classic symptom is coughing with difficulty producing any sputum and high fever. The lateral chest X-ray is usually definitive and shows an irregular tracheal wall. High-dose intravenous antibiotics and cool mist oxygen via a mask are the appropriate treatments. Bronchoscopic debridement is not necessary and is contraindicated as it will inevitably cause diffuse bleeding and distress.

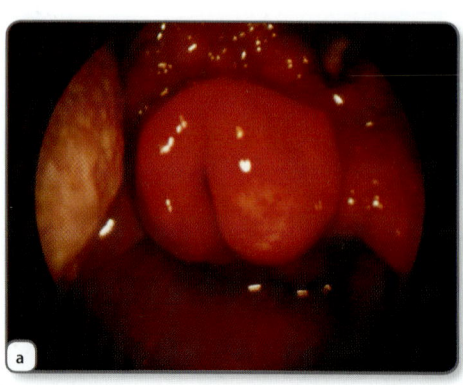

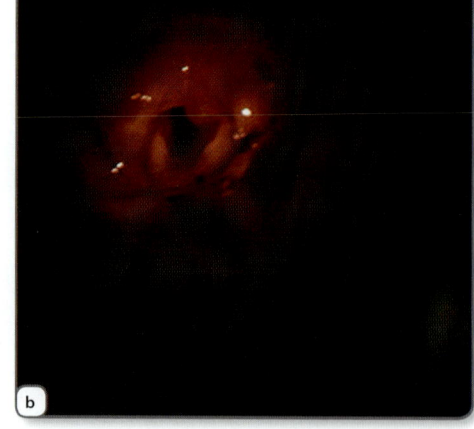

Figure 9.19 (a and b) Examples of acute epiglottitis.

Neck abscesses

Neck abscesses can be so large as to be obstructive. If present in the young infant, an immune deficiency is possible. Compression can be relieved by needle aspiration prior to intubation if the child is in distress. Incision and drainage is required with appropriate antibiotics (Vieira et al. 2008). Some neck infections travel down the great vessels into the mediastinum, producing mediastinitis and massive pleural effusions, and thus cause compromise of the airway. Thoracotomy and pleural decortication are frequently required as well. Mediastinitis is frequently fatal despite treatment (**Figure 9.20**).

Necrotizing fasciitis

Necrotizing fasciitis is a massive tissue destructive infection with anaerobes and facultative anaerobes. It usually involves the deep neck spaces and rarely involves the larynx or trachea. Aggressive wide excision of the involved skin, muscles, and adipose tissue is required, but conservative debridement of the adjacent laryngeal and tracheal tissue is usually adequate, preserving the recurrent nerves and vasculature. High-dose appropriate antibiotics are necessary, and hyperbaric oxygen treatments are beneficial. Tracheotomy may be required.

Iatrogenic injury

Iatrogenic injury to the airway is not uncommon. Lasers function at high temperatures and are a common cause of injury to the airway. An operator not familiar with the proper power or duration of the beam pulse energy can burn tissues too deeply or too widely. Perhaps, the most devastating catastrophe with a laser is a fire during carbon

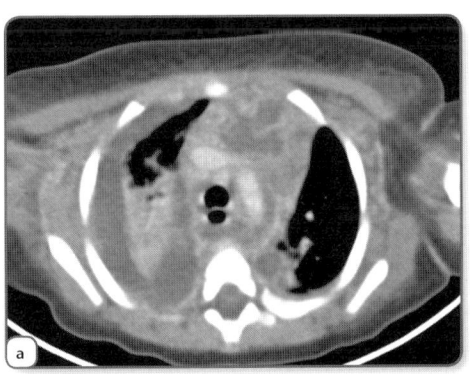
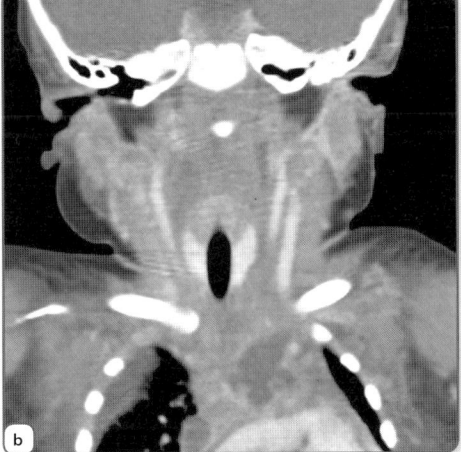

Figure 9.20 Mediastinitis (a) axial and (b) coronal views.

dioxide (CO_2) laser endoscopy. The entire airway from the oropharynx to the distal bronchi can be injured, and sometimes even the skin. Appropriate caution followed by the use of low oxygen concentrations, low laser power, and using a pulse mode rather than continuous delivery can diminish the likelihood of a fire. Treatment is to stop the laser, turn off the oxygen supply, and begin ventilating with room air. If an endotracheal tube or tracheostomy tube was in the field of the laser, it should be removed as well in case it has ignited. Re-endoscopy should be performed to evaluate the extent of the injury, and the administration of steroids and antibiotics should be started. Fires have also been reported during electrocautery tracheotomy and tonsillectomy. The flame is invisible, and sometimes the first hint of a fire is the melting of the surgeon's glove and the subsequent perceived heat and pain (Thompson et al. 1998). Again, the first treatment is to turn off the cautery, smother the flame with a wet drape, remove any plastic tubes from the field, ventilate with room air, start antibiotic and steroid administration, and undertake a formal endoscopy of the airway. Multiple failed attempts to intubate can leave the larynx swollen and bloody, making intubation difficult. Recurrent nerve injury has been reported from failed intubation attempts. Choosing a bronchoscope that is too big can precipitate an emergent tracheotomy by producing swelling in a narrow subglottic region. Familiarity with the relevant anatomy, knowing the limit of one's skills, and possessing enough experience to know the correct size of instruments to use in all cases can usually prevent significant damage to the airway and unnecessary tracheotomies. Balloon dilation injuries are more frequent and a death has been reported, though most are handled by observation. The back wall of the trachea has been inadvertently cut and the esophagus entered during emergent tracheotomy without sequelae. Once recognized and repaired with interrupted simple 6–0 silk sutures and nasogastric feeding, the injury heals without stricture or symptoms. Bleeding from too vigorous a bronchoscopy in the distal bronchi is managed with a pseudoephedrine solution instilled into the airway and then suctioned out. This procedure is repeated until the bleeding subsides.

Post-tonsillectomy hemorrhage and scarring

Unfortunately, post-tonsillectomy hemorrhage is a common event and a challenge for the anesthesiologist. The patient must be taken to the operating room and given a general anesthetic on a full stomach while the airway is being flooded with blood from the lateral pharyngeal wall. A rapid sequence intravenous agent technique is required, with cricoid pressure. Once the patient is intubated and the airway is secured, the surgeon can stop the bleeding. Excessive use of cautery current can cause severe nasopharyngeal and pharyngeal scarring, which requires extensive reconstructive surgery (**Figure 9.21**).

Treatment options include endoscopic excision, marsupialization, and laser ablation. Recurrence is fairly common, rendering surveillance necessary. Saccular cysts are less common than ductal cysts and present earlier with more severe airway compromise. Saccular cysts are described as dilated, mucus-filled saccules of the laryngeal ventricle. Lateral saccular cysts are most common and may extend laterally via the thyrohyoid membrane into the neck. Diagnosis involves FFL and direct laryngoscopy. Treatment may occur via endoscopic marsupialization, laser excision, or transcervical approaches for large or recurrent saccular cysts. Postoperative observation is important, as recurrence is known to occur.

Hemangiomas

Hemangiomas are the most common pediatric head and neck neoplasm, but constitute only 1% of congenital laryngeal neoplasms. The natural course of hemangiomas is a rapid proliferation stage over the first year of life followed by an involution stage over the next 10–12 years (Ida et al. 2008). Women are twice as likely to be afflicted as men. The etiology is thought to involve mesodermal rests of vasoformative tissue. Patients often present in the first 8 weeks to 6 months of life with biphasic stridor, intermittent respiratory distress, croup-like coughing, and feeding difficulties. Of patients with airway hemangiomas, 50% have other cutaneous hemangiomas. Diagnosis is made by history, physical examination, direct laryngoscopy, and bronchoscopy. The hemangioma most often appears as a unilateral, single sessile, compressible, bluish-pink mass in the subglottis (**Figure 8.10**). After diagnosis, some advocate for an MRI to detect extralaryngeal and intracranial hemangiomas (Javia et al. 2011). As spontaneous regression is possible, observation may be possible for very small hemangiomas, but careful observation is necessary. There are a variety of medical, endoscopic, and open techniques available to manage laryngeal hemangiomas. Propranolol, a nonselective β-2 antagonist,

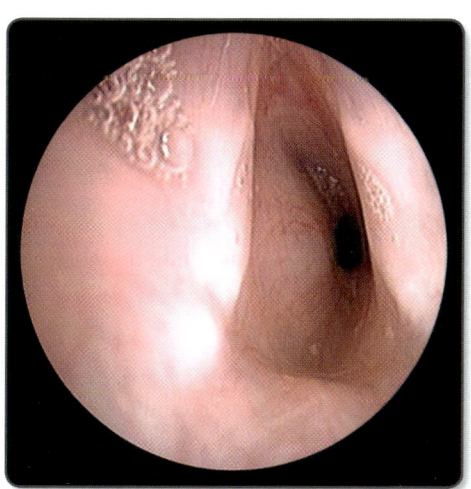

Figure 8.10 Endoscopic view showing a unilateral, smooth swelling in the subglottis, the classical appearance of a subglottic hemangioma. With permission from Bajaj Y, Kapoor K, Ifeacho S, et al. Great Ormond Street Hospital treatment guidelines for use of propranolol in infantile isolated subglottic haemangioma. J Laryngol Otol 2013; 127:295–298.

has demonstrated efficacy in producing hemangioma regression. There are cardiovascular risks associated with its use, of which hypotension, bradycardia, and hypoglycemia are the most prominent ones (Bajaj et al. 2013). Electrocardiogram and echocardiogram, as well as an extensive history and physical examination, are performed prior to its use. Propranolol is often used over a course of 12 months, with serial endoscopic evaluations used to assess hemangioma regression. The Great Ormond Street Hospital in London has published its protocol (**Figure 8.11**). Other treatment modalities include steroids (systemic or intralesional), laser endoscopic ablation, open resection, and, in severe cases, tracheostomy with observation. Long-term follow-up of hemagioma patients is advocated.

Stenosis

Congenital laryngotracheal stenosis (LTS) is a less common cause of neonatal stridor. The majority of LTS is acquired from etiologies, such as intubation trauma, caustic ingestion, and GERD. Failure of the recanalization process during fetal airway embryogenesis is thought to produce congenital airway stenosis (**Figure 8.12**). Complete atresia may occur and requires management with an ex utero intrapartum treatment (EXIT) procedure. Congenital LTS is often associated with syndromes such as 22q11 deletion, CHARGE, trisomy 21, and Fraser (Blanchard et al. 2013). Patients with LTS present with stridor within the first few weeks of life, a croup-like cough, and hoarse cry. If the stenosis is severe, then the patient may present with respiratory distress. Diagnosis is made by endoscopic evaluation of the laryngotracheal tree. Subglottic stenosis is defined by a subglottic diameter <4 mm in a

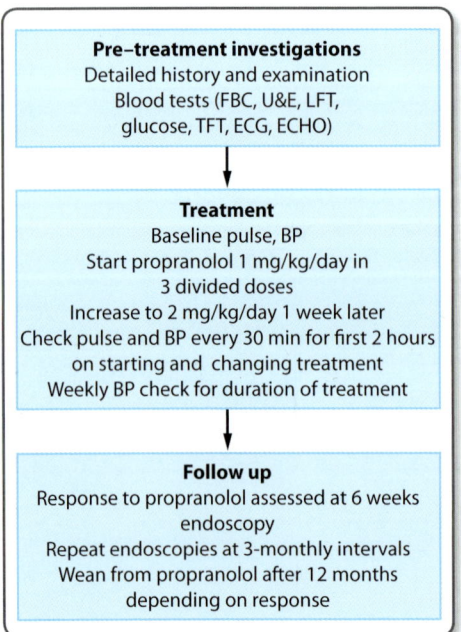

Pre–treatment investigations
Detailed history and examination
Blood tests (FBC, U&E, LFT,
glucose, TFT, ECG, ECHO)

Treatment
Baseline pulse, BP
Start propranolol 1 mg/kg/day in
3 divided doses
Increase to 2 mg/kg/day 1 week later
Check pulse and BP every 30 min for first 2 hours
on starting and changing treatment
Weekly BP check for duration of treatment

Follow up
Response to propranolol assessed at 6 weeks
endoscopy
Repeat endoscopies at 3-monthly intervals
Wean from propranolol after 12 months
depending on response

Figure 8.11 Flow chart for propranolol treatment for infantile subglottic hemangioma. FBC, full blood count; U&E, urea and electrolyte analysis; LFT, liver function tests; TFT, thyroid function tests; ECG, electrocardiography; ECHO, echocardiography; BP, blood pressure. With permission from Bajaj Y, Kapoor K, Ifeacho S, et al. Great Ormond Street Hospital treatment guidelines for use of propranolol in infantile isolated subglottic haemangioma. J Laryngol Otol 2013; 127:295–298.

Plastic bronchitis

The Fontan cardiac operation drastically alters the pressure gradients of the lungs. This allows the transudation of proteins from the blood into the bronchial lumens where they solidify into an elastic compound that forms 'casts' and obstructs the airway, known as plastic bronchitis (Quasney et al. 2000). The best way to manage these casts is to hydraulically flush them out by placing a small catheter distal to the cast and forcefully irrigating to mobilize them outward, and then removing them mechanically with forceps through rigid bronchoscopy. Once they have been removed, urokinase instillation can prevent their reformation by liquefying the material as it crosses the alveolar membranes (**Figure 9.22**).

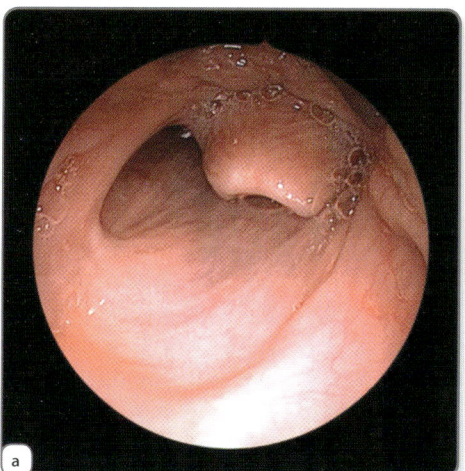 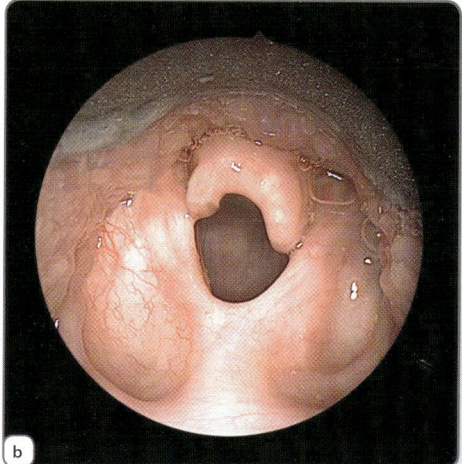

Figure 9.21 (a and b) Pharyngeal cautery scars.

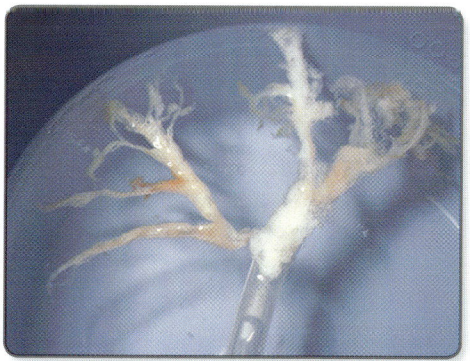

Figure 9.22 Plastic bronchitis.

Pediatric tracheotomy

The timing of a pediatric tracheotomy is critical. Optimization of certain criteria should be sought. All pediatric tracheotomies should be done in the operating room. The patient must be stable enough to tolerate a brief apnea while hemostasis is being achieved with an electric cautery and while the endotracheal tube is being removed and the tracheostomy tube is inserted. High oxygen concentrations should be avoided. The peak inspiratory ventilation pressures must not exceed 35 cmH$_2$O because the neonatal high compliance cuff will leak at pressures above that level, and the patient cannot be adequately ventilated, no matter how much water or air is passed into the cuff. High compliance cuffs should be used to prevent tracheal mucosa damage from high cuff pressures that are compounded by the addition of ventilator pressures. Ventilator settings can be modified to deliver larger volumes over a long inspiration, or more frequent shorter breaths to drop the peak inspiratory pressure, depending on the pulmonary status. Tight to shaft cuffs are preferable, so that a smaller tracheotomy hole can be used, and thus less damage caused to the trachea. Other cuffs are bulky even when deflated, making them more difficult to insert in small babies, even with the use of lubrication. Patients should be >1200 g in weight so that a 2.5 mm or 3.0 mm neonatal tracheostomy tube will be short enough not to touch the carina and cause bradycardia or irritation. The 2.5 mm lumens are so small that they are difficult to keep open and require an inordinate amount of care. The primary cause of tracheostomy-related death immediately after surgery is accidental decannulation, when the tracheostomy tube falls out and on reinsertion passes into the mediastinum. Creating a superior and inferior tracheal flap sewn to the skin, called a Bjork flap, can prevent this problem (**Figures 9.23** and **9.24**). The trachea is cut in an 'H' fashion instead of the classical vertical incision. Sewing flaps to the skin is called maturing the stoma and makes it difficult for the tracheostomy tube to fail to enter the trachea. In addition, the tracheostomy tube flanges can be sewn to the skin in a four-quadrant fashion for 1 week until the tracheostomy track fully matures (**Figure 9.25**). At the authors' institution, a double Bjork flap and flange stitches have been used, with no 'false passages' and no immediate postoperative tracheostomy-related deaths in >400 patients. Infants have higher normal coagulation studies than older children, but they still bleed more easily at surgery. Normalization of the values to the pediatric normal for 24 hours with fresh frozen plasma is beneficial and presents no greater risks.

Conclusion

Managing the pediatric airway can be difficult due to the small sizes and the extremely small margins for error. Rapid correct evaluation of the patient's status, the use of proper equipment, the presence of well-trained support staff, an appropriate facility, and the skill of the

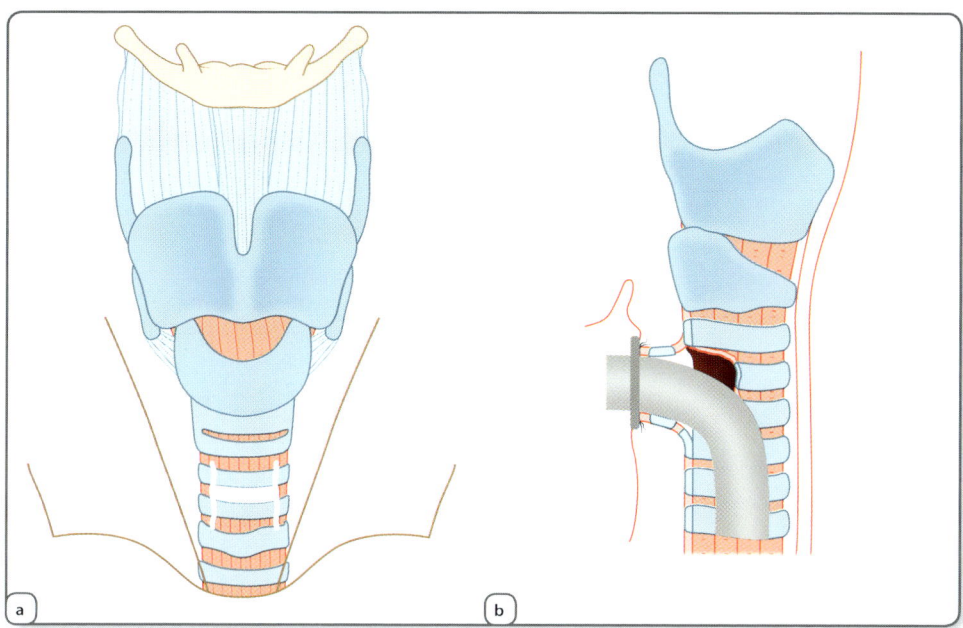

Figure 9.23 Bjork flap. (a) Anterior and (b) sagittal views.

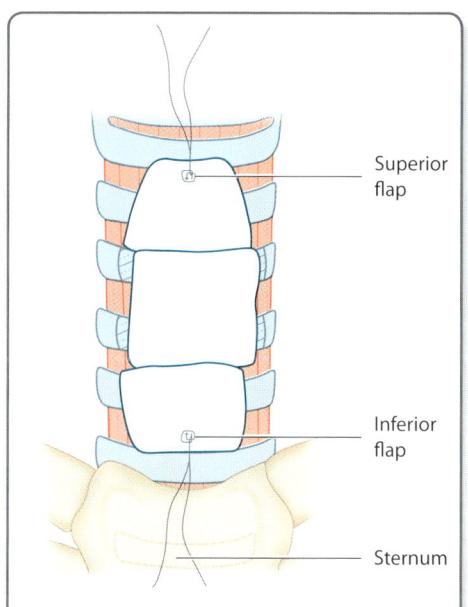

Superior flap

Inferior flap

Sternum

Figure 9.24 Bjork flap lateral.

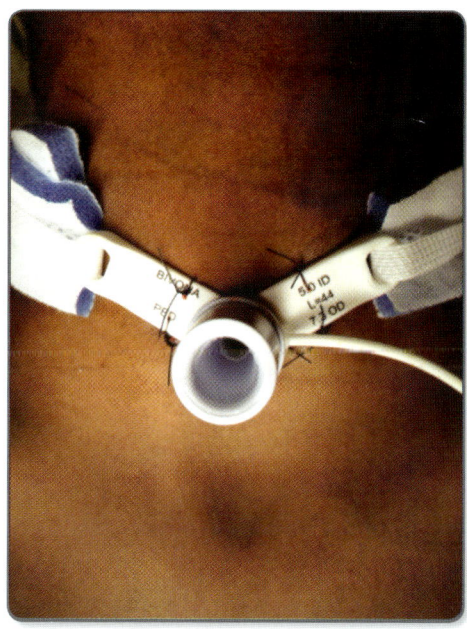

Figure 9.25 Tracheostomy tube flange sewn into position.

surgeon are all critical factors in obtaining a good outcome. Knowledge is the single most important tool a surgeon must have. When blended with skill, experience, and the proper setting, the patients benefit.

References

Busch RF, Shah D. Ludwig's angina: improved treatment. Otolaryngol Head Neck Surg 1997; 117:172–175.

Ladurner R, Qvick LM, Hohenbleicher F, et al. Pneumopericardium in blunt chest trauma after high-speed motor vehicle accidents. Am J Emerg Med 2005; 23:83–86.

Quasney MW, Orman K, Thompson JW, et al. Plastic bronchitis later after Fontan procedure: treatment with aerosolized urokinase. Crit Care Med 2000; 28:2107–2111.

Rashid M, Karagama Y. Inflation of Foley catheters for postnasal packing. J Laryngol Otol 2010; 124:997–998.

Robinson L, Miller R. Smoke inhalation injuries. Am J Otolaryngol 1986; 7:375–380.

Stack BC Jr., Ridley MB. Arytenoid subluxation from blunt laryngeal trauma. Am J Otolaryngol 1994; 15:68–73.

Shafer SD, Brown OE. Selective application of CT in the management of laryngeal trauma. Laryngoscope 1983; 93:1473–1475.

Thompson JW, Colin W, Snowden T, et al. Fire in the operating room during tracheostomy. South Med J 1998; 91:243–247.

Vieira F, Allen SM, Stocks RM, Thompson JW. Deep neck infection. Otolaryngol Clin North Am 2008; 41:459–483.

Zur KB, Litman RS. Pediatric airway foreign body retrieval: surgical and anesthetic perspectives. Paediatr Anesth 2009; 19:109–117.

Further reading

Bluestone C. Pediatric Otolaryngology, 4th edn. Philadelphia: Saunders, 2001.

Bradley NJ, Darling JL, Oktar N, et al. The failure of human leukocyte interferon to influence the growth of human glioma cell populations: in vitro and in vivo studies. Br J Cancer 1983; 48:819-825.

King C, Henrelig FM. Pediatric emergency procedures. Philadelphia: Lippincott Williams & Wilkins, 2008.

Ossoff RO (ed.). The Larynx. Philadelphia: Lippincott Williams & Wilkins, 2003.

Rovin JD, Rodgers BM. Pediatric foreign body aspiration. Pediatric Rev 2000; 21:86-90.

10 The EXIT procedure

Rose Mary Stocks, Jonathan P Giurintano

History

Originating from a series of experimental fetal operations on primates began in 1982 by Michael Harrison and colleagues at the University of California, San Francisco, ex utero intrapartum therapy (the EXIT procedure) introduced a novel mechanism for correcting congenital malformations in utero (Harrison et al. 1982). Prior to these experiments, fetal surgery incurred high rates of mortality, as attempted manipulation of the exquisitely sensitive human uterus rapidly leads to induction of preterm labor and fetal demise, but Harrison's work laid the foundation for the anesthetic and surgical approaches and tocolytic management of both the mother and the fetus.

Designed on the principle of operating on a partially-delivered fetus still connected to the maternal circulation, the EXIT procedure was initially used in the treatment of congenital disorders such as urogenital obstruction and diaphragmatic hernia, only later gaining popularity for the management of congenital head and neck masses. Use of the EXIT procedure in pediatric anesthesia and otolaryngology was first reported in 1989 at Thomas Jefferson University in an attempt to secure airway access in a fetus with a large cervical teratoma obstructing the airway. Norris and colleagues attempted to gain airway access while maintaining placental circulation for 10 minutes by rigid bronchoscopy and tracheotomy, but their attempts were unsuccessful and the neonate died during the procedure (Norris et al. 1989). In 1992 Langer and associates reported the first successful intubation using the EXIT procedure in a fetus with an obstructing anterior cervical teratoma, though several hours later the fetus expired due to pharyngeal hemorrhage and dislodgement of the endotracheal tube (Langer et al. 1992). As surgical and anesthetic techniques continued to be refined throughout the 1990s, the EXIT procedure emerged as a valuable mechanism for securing airway access in neonates with a broad range of congenital malformations that place the fetus at risk of severe hypoxia or a fatal outcome at birth.

Pharmacologic and fetal theories of the EXIT procedure

Fetal physiology

As the chief principle of the EXIT procedure is maintenance of maternal–fetal circulation, an understanding of the fetal circulatory system is a prerequisite for understanding the purpose of the EXIT procedure. Unlike the adult, the fetal respiratory system provides little function, with gas exchange occurring via the placenta rather than the medical, bioethical, and psychosocial care, informed consent for the procedure is obtained, and a multidisciplinary team is assembled. The average gestational age for a fetus undergoing the EXIT procedure is 34 weeks (Marwan & Crombleholme 2006).

The team

It must be stressed that the EXIT procedure involves two patients – the mother and the fetus – both of whom are at high risk of morbidity and mortality, and in order to ensure a successful procedure, a multidisciplinary team of health-care professionals should be assembled at the onset of procedure planning. Representatives from radiology, obstetrics and maternal–fetal medicine, pediatric surgery, otolaryngology, pediatric and obstetric anesthesiology, neonatology, nursing, and medical ethics should be called to review the case. With the team assembled, an appropriate operating room should be identified, the layout of the room and location of each team's position and surgical equipment designated, and the actual steps of the procedure and management plans should be practiced multiple times. The layout should be designed so that the obstetric surgeon and otolaryngologist can work simultaneously, with the obstetrician partially delivering the fetus and preventing placental separation while the otolaryngologist secures the airway. Operating room layout will be institution-specific, but a single large operating room or two smaller adjacent operating rooms must be available in the event that the neonate requires immediate surgery postdelivery [e.g. mass excision or extracorporeal membrane oxygenation (ECMO)] (**Table 10.1**).

Radiology

Planning for the EXIT procedure begins with the evaluation of fetal position and placental location, for which a portable ultrasound machine should be present. The ideal position for the EXIT procedure is for the fetus to be located in a cephalic position with the neck in extension. The optimal hysterotomy incision may be located by

Table 10.1 Recommended equipment for the EXIT procedure
Portable ultrasound machine
Laryngoscope handle
Miller 00, 0, and 1 blades
Endotracheal tubes (sizes 2.5, 3.0, 3.5, 4.0 mm)
2.5 mm rigid bronchoscope with 0 degree lens
Endoscopy video tower and light source
Tracheostomy tray
Tracheostomy tubes (sizes 3.0, 3.5, 4.0 mm)
Bipolar and monopolar electrocautery
Suction equipment

mapping the placental edges using ultrasound. The procedure may be performed even if the fetus is in an alternate position, but the incision may have to be extended to achieve adequate exposure of the head and neck. Additionally, ultrasonography allows the team to evaluate the lesion's location as well as its vascularity. Characterization of the lesion's vascularity is important because a fetus with a highly vascular lesion may quickly decompensate once the cord is severed, even if the procedure is successful. Cystic masses can be decompressed percutaneously prior to the procedure, improving the chances of airway access and minimizing the extent of uterine incision, thus decreasing maternal morbidity (Dighe et al. 2011).

Maternal anesthesia

With the fetal location known and the mass characterized, attention should then turn to placing the mother under general anesthesia. Goals for the mother include:

1. Adequate general anesthesia for the mother without recall
2. Maximal uterine relaxation to facilitate delivery of the fetal head while minimizing the chance of placental detachment

As previously discussed, a successful EXIT procedure requires uterine relaxation, maintenance of uterine volume, and prevention of neonatal respiration to delay placental detachment. Standard rapid-sequence inhalation agents are used, with intravenous nitroglycerin or terbutaline to maintain uterine relaxation, and the patient is placed either supine with left uterine displacement or in the left lateral decubitus position. At least 20 minutes of general anesthesia is administered to allow for adequate uterine relaxation prior to incision. Anesthesia is maintained with halothane, isoflurane, or sevoflurane in 50% oxygen, often with additional intravenous sedation including fentanyl.

Pediatric anesthesia

Fetal anesthesia is largely maintained with maternal inhalational anesthetic passing through the uteroplacental circulation. However, as complete fetal paralysis is critical to prevent fetal respiration and facilitate manipulation as the otolaryngologist is obtaining airway access, additional intramuscular fetal paralytics and narcotics are often administered through the deltoid muscle. A pulse oximetry probe and fetal scalp electrode monitor should also be connected for monitoring of fetal oxygen saturation and pulse during the procedure.

Obstetrics and maternal–fetal medicine

With the mother and fetus under general anesthesia, the maternal abdominal cavity can be entered. Although a standard Pfannenstiel incision is typically adequate, exposure of the uterus is critical, and the possibility of entry via a vertical abdominal incision should not be dismissed because of decreased postoperative cosmesis. Initially, a hysterotomy incision of only 2 cm is made with a scalpel; the incision is then extended to the degree necessary for delivery of the fetal neck and head using a special hysterotomy stapler that maintains hemostasis of the cut uterine edges while the fetus is being treated. With the uterus open, only the fetal head and neck as well as one extremity, are delivered in order to minimize fetal heat loss and to decrease the risk of umbilical cord compromise or premature placental detachment.

Pediatric otolaryngology

With the head and neck exposed, attention may be turned to securing the neonate's airway. With good anesthesia, maternal–fetal circulation can typically be maintained for at least 60 minutes, affording the otolaryngologist sufficient time to gain airway access (Liechty et al. 1997). With a Miller blade laryngoscope, direct laryngoscopy may initially be performed. If the laryngeal inlet is easily visualized with direct laryngoscopy, orotracheal intubation should be attempted to gain airway access. If this is unsuccessful, or if the laryngeal inlet is difficult to visualize with direct laryngoscopy, fiberoptic endotracheal intubation may be attempted. If airway access is still inaccessible or there is no visualization of the larynx on direct laryngoscopy, rigid bronchoscopy and tracheostomy, with or without excision of the mass or drainage of the cyst, can be performed while the fetus is maintained on the maternal uteroplacental circulation (**Figure 10.2**).

Neonatology

With the fetal airway secured, the umbilical cord is then clamped and cut. The intubated neonate is handed to the neonatologist and taken to the growing table for assessment and further resuscitation. It must be recalled that because the fetus is under the effects of general anesthesia and neuromuscular blocking agents, the Apgar scores obtained immediately after delivery should be inaccurately low. With the fetus safely delivered, uterine relaxation is rapidly reversed to prevent maternal hemorrhage from uterine hypotonia. The uterus is rapidly closed, the mother's general anesthesia is reversed and she is taken to the postanesthesia care unit.

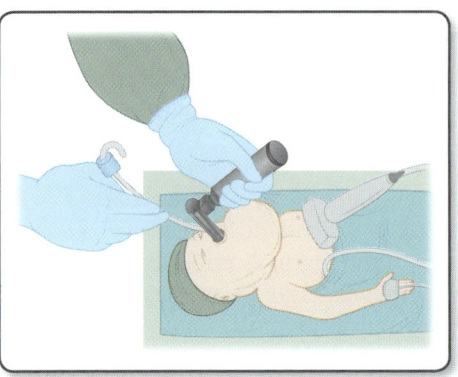

Figure 10.2 Delivery via the EXIT procedure.

The operating room should be designed so that the obstetrician and otolaryngologist can work in coordination, the obstetrician performing the hysterostomy and otolaryngologist securing the airway, after which the umbilical cord is severed and the infant is passed to the neonatology team. A separate operating area should be prepared in case the infant requires further surgical intervention immediately after placental detachment.

Potential complications and strategies

Although in most cases, airway access may be obtained through direct laryngoscopy, bronchoscopy, or tracheostomy, there is the potential that a fetus may have an anterior neck mass that precludes airway access from being obtained at the time of the EXIT procedure. In this case (**Table 10.2**), ECMO may be required to maintain oxygenation in the neonate. ECMO involves extravascular cannulation of the internal carotid artery and internal jugular vein, and may be instituted while the fetus is receiving placental oxygenation so that before the umbilical cord is severed, the fetus is bridged to extracorporeal oxygenation, avoiding hypercapnea or anoxic injury until definitive access can be obtained (Ortiz et al. 1987). Infants younger than 35 weeks are not candidates for ECMO because of a high incidence of intracranial hemorrhage, but EXIT-to-ECMO remains a viable option in fetuses older than 35 weeks who are unable to initially undergo tracheostomy.

Conclusion

Prior to the advent of the EXIT procedure in the 1980s, births of fetuses with congenital abnormalities causing airway obstruction carried severely high rates of mortality. It has been estimated that the mortality

Table 10.2 Congenital head and neck anomalies warranting the EXIT procedure
Cystic lymphatic malformation
Cervical teratoma
Micrognathia
Congenital cystic adenomatoid malformation
Epignathic tumor
Hemangioma
Congenital goiter
Choristoma
Neuroblastoma
Granular cell tumor
Retinoblastoma
Mucocele
Branchial cleft cyst
Laryngocele

of newborns with a cervical mass before the advent of the EXIT procedure was up to 40% (Jordan & Gauderer 1988). If the airway is not secured within 5 minutes following termination of maternal–fetal circulation, anoxic brain injury will result. In order for a procedure to be successful, the surgeon must understand the underlying maternal and fetal physiology, a multidisciplinary approach must be taken by physicians and nurses from a range of medical specialties, and there must be a well-practiced, seamless institution of the procedure in the operating room to ensure the safety of both the infant and mother.

References

Dighe M, Peterson S, Dubinsky T, et al. EXIT procedure: technique and indications with prenatal imaging parameters for assessment of airway patency. RadioGraphics 2011; 31:511–526.

Gundry SR, Wesley JR, Klein MD, et al. Cervical teratomas in the newborn. JPediatr Surg 1983; 18:382–386.

Harrison MR, Anderson J, Rosen MA, et al. Fetal surgery in the primate I. Anesthetic, surgical, and tocolytic management to maximize fetal-neonatal survival. J Pediatr Surg 1982; 17:115–122.

Jordan RB, Gauderer MW. Cervical teratomas: an analysis. Literature review and proposed classification. J Pediatr Surg 1988; 23:583–591.

Lake CL. Cardiac embryology, growth, and development. In: Lake CL (ed.), Pediatric cardiac anesthesia. East Norwalk, CT: Appleton & Lange, 1988:27–42.

Langer JC, Tabb T, Thompson P, et al. Management of prenatally diagnosed tracheal obstruction: access to the airway in utero prior to delivery. Fetal Diagn Ther 1992; 7:12–16.

Liechty KW, Crombleholme TM, Flake AW, et al. Intrapartum airway management for giant fetal neck masses: the EXIT (ex utero intrapartum treatment) procedure. Am J Obstet Gynecol 1997; 177:870–874.

Marwan A, Crombleholme TM. The EXIT procedure: principles, pitfalls, and progress. Semin Pediatr Surg 2006; 15:107–115.

Meschia G. Placental respiratory gas exchange and fetal oxygenation. In: Creasy RK, Resnik R (eds), Maternal-fetal medicine principles and practice, 3rd edn. Philadelphia, PA: WB Saunders Co, 1994:288–294.

Norris MC, Joseph J, Leighton BL. Anesthesia for perinatal surgery. Am J Perinatol 1989; 6:39–40.

Ortiz RM, Cilley RE, Bartlett RH. Extracorporeal membrane oxygenation in pediatric respiratory failure. Pediatr Clin North Am 1987; 34:39–46.

Schwartz M, Tashijian W, Parker M, et al. Anesthetic management of the exit (ex utero intrapartum treatment) procedure. J Clin Anesth 2001; 13(5):387–391.

Further reading

Bouchard S, Johnson M, Flake A, et al. The EXIT procedure: experience and outcome in 31 cases. J Pediatr Surg 2002; 37(3):418–426.

Stocks, RM, Egerman R, Woodson G, et al. Airway management of neonates with antenatally detected head and neck anomalies. Arch Otolaryngol Head Neck Surg 1997; 123:641–645.

Taghavi, K, Beasley, S. The ex utero intrapartum treatment (EXIT) procedure: application of a new therapeutic paradigm. J Paediatr Child Health 2013; 49:420–427.

Reconstruction of the airway

Catherine K Hart, Christina J Yang, Michael J Rutter

Introduction

The introduction of laryngotracheoplasty in the 1970s paved the way for surgical innovations and continued progress in airway reconstruction over the next several decades. By the early 2000s, expansion and resection techniques had become the cornerstone of the open surgical management of pediatric laryngotracheal stenosis. At present, the slide tracheoplasty is gaining acceptance and has become a valuable addition to the surgical armamentarium. This chapter presents an overview of preoperative patient assessment and optimization and subsequently outlines current approaches to operative management.

Preoperative evaluation and optimization

The importance of carrying out a thorough preoperative evaluation and ensuring patient optimization cannot be overemphasized, as both are essential to successful surgical outcomes. In many clinical settings, this evaluation is collaboratively undertaken by an interdisciplinary team composed of experts in pulmonology, gastroenterology, otolaryngology, and speech pathology (**Table 11.1**). To evaluate vocal fold function, all children should undergo flexible laryngoscopy. It is also useful to assess swallowing function and the risk of aspiration by performing both a videofluoroscopic swallow study and a fiberoptic endoscopic evaluation of swallowing (Willging 2000, Hartnick et al. 2000). Given that gastroesophageal reflux disease, eosinophilic esophagitis, an 'active' larynx, and airway colonization

Table 11.1 Components of preoperative evaluation prior to open airway procedure

Diagnostic test/procedure	Goal of test
Microlaryngoscopy, bronchoscopy	Assess airway and characterize stenosis
Flexible bronchoscopy	Assess airway dynamics and pulmonary comorbidities
EGD with biopsies	Assess gastrointestinal tract, rule out eosinophilic esophagitis
pH-multichannel impedance testing	Assess for gastroesophageal reflux
VSS +/– FEES	Determine safety of swallow, assess for aspiration
Flexible laryngoscopy Tracheal and nasal cultures	Evaluate vocal fold function Rule out MRSA and/or pseudomonas colonization

EGD, esophagogastroduodenoscopy; FEES, fiberoptic endoscopic evaluation of swallowing; MRSA, methicillin-resistant *Staphylococcus aureus*; VSS, videofluoroscopic swallow study.

with pseudomonas or methicillin-resistant *Staphylococcus aureus* are all conditions known to have a negative impact on surgical success, these conditions should be diagnosed and addressed prior to surgical intervention (White et al. 2005, de Alarcon & Rutter 2008, Meier & White 2012, Statham et al. 2012).

Careful and thorough endoscopic evaluation of the airway to assess the grade, severity, and location of the stenosis is imperative. This allows for the identification of secondary airway lesions, which may influence the surgeon's decision regarding the operation selected. Microlaryngoscopy is performed to examine the supraglottis and glottis. The supraglottis is assessed for laryngomalacia and stenosis, and the glottis is assessed for stenosis, posterior glottis stenosis, anterior glottic web, and laryngeal cleft. If vocal fold immobility is suspected, the cricoarytenoid joints should be palpated to assess for joint fixation.

Rigid bronchoscopy is performed using a Hopkins rod telescope and/or a rigid bronchoscope. The subglottis is evaluated. If stenosis is present, the extent of the narrowing is determined using endotracheal tubes and then classified using the Myer–Cotton scale. The length of the stenosis and its proximity to the vocal folds are also determined. If a tracheotomy is present, evaluation of the suprastomal area for suprastomal collapse, granuloma, or an intratracheal skin tract is performed. The remainder of the trachea down to the carina is assessed for additional airway pathology, including tracheal stenosis, complete tracheal rings, tracheoesophageal fistula (TEF), residual TEF pouch, vascular compression, and tracheomalacia.

Preoperative planning

Single- versus double-stage procedures

Airway reconstruction can be performed either as a single- or double-stage procedure. In a single-stage procedure, the airway is reconstructed without placement of a tracheostomy or with removal of the tracheostomy at the time of the reconstruction. In a double-stage procedure, the existing tracheostomy remains in place or a tracheostomy is performed at the beginning of the reconstruction. Multiple factors influence the surgeon's decision as to whether to perform a single- or double-stage reconstruction. These factors include the surgeon's comfort level with the procedure, the capability of the intensive care unit to manage the patient postoperatively, the severity of the stenosis, and the severity of the patient's medical comorbidities. Patients with poor pulmonary function, multilevel airway obstruction, a known history of difficult intubation, a history of sedation issues, or previous reconstructive failure are considered poor candidates for single-stage reconstruction.

In a single-stage procedure, the patient is usually nasally intubated for a period as brief as a few hours to as long as 2 weeks. The duration of intubation depends on the procedure performed (**Table 11.2**). In some cases, a single-stage procedure provides significant benefit. For

Table 11.2 Intubation guidelines for single-stage procedures	
Procedure	Duration of intubation (days)
Anterior costal cartilage graft	0–5
Posterior costal cartilage graft	5–10
Anterior and posterior costal cartilage grafts	7–14
Cricotracheal resection	0–5
Tracheal resection	0–5
Slide tracheoplasty	0–3

example, in a child with stenosis associated with the tracheostoma, the risk of postoperative recurrence is minimized if the tracheostomy is removed at the time of reconstruction. Although a single-stage procedure offers advantages such as the avoidance of a tracheostomy or immediate decannulation, it is also associated with risks. One of the most significant risks is unplanned extubation. To mitigate this risk, many patients, particularly those <3 years of age, receive heavy sedation. In turn, sedation increases the risk of pulmonary complications and hypotension requiring inotropic support (McCormick et al. 2013). Older patients often tolerate intubation with little or no sedation, and some are able to ambulate and eat while intubated.

In most double-stage procedures, a stent is placed to support the reconstructed area. The position and duration of stenting depend upon the reconstruction performed. If a reconstruction involves the subglottis, a suprastomal stent is positioned with the distal end just above the tracheostomy and the proximal end lying at the level of the false vocal folds. To minimize the risk of aspiration, the proximal end of the stent is either capped or sewn shut. Although a silicone stent is generally preferred, a cut T-tube or Teflon stent can also be used (Preciado 2012). Children with suprastomal stents in place are essentially tracheostomy tube-dependent, making accidental decannulation a potentially catastrophic event.

Endoscopic surgery

Advancements in the design of endoscopic instruments over the last decade have played an important role in the resurgence of endoscopic airway management. Endoscopic techniques can be used both as the primary treatment modality in properly selected patients and as an adjuvant treatment following open airway reconstruction. Patients with straightforward grade 1 or grade 2 stenosis and no history of previous endoscopic failure have a higher likelihood of successful endoscopic management. Those with grade 3 or grade 4 stenosis or multilevel stenoses are more likely to require an open reconstruction (Simpson et al. 1982). Specific endoscopic surgical techniques are discussed elsewhere in this text.

Expansion surgery

The goal of expansion surgery is not to excise tissue, but rather to augment the airway by inserting grafts to expand the airway lumen.

Graft materials

Costal cartilage

Costal cartilage is the most commonly used graft material, as it is readily available and is easily carved into the appropriate shape. An additional advantage is that more than one graft can be harvested through a single incision, which is usually placed over the right fifth or sixth rib. In girls, the incision is placed in the anticipated breast crease for cosmetic reasons. The incision is carried down through the subcutaneous tissue and muscle. A self-retaining retractor is placed to facilitate exposure, and the superior and inferior muscular attachments are divided. The perichondrium is carefully incised along the superior and inferior edges of the rib to identify the subperichondrial plane. A Freer elevator is used to separate the perichondrium from the posterior surface of the rib. Once this plane has been identified, a Doyen periosteal elevator can be used to completely separate the rib from the perichondrium. A 30-gauge needle is used to identify the osteocartilaginous junction, and a scalpel is used to divide the rib at this junction, cutting down onto the Doyen elevator to protect the underlying pleura. The graft is then elevated off the perichondrium from lateral to medial and divided at the sternal margin. The wound is then filled with saline, and a Valsalva maneuver is performed to confirm that the pleura has not been violated. The wound is closed in layers over a Penrose drain. The graft is carved to the desired shape with the perichondrium facing the lumen of the airway.

Thyroid ala cartilage

Thyroid ala cartilage is utilized when only a small graft is required. It is harvested from the superior aspect of the thyroid cartilage, at least 1 mm above the level of the true vocal folds. Thyroid ala can be quickly and easily harvested without the need for an additional incision; however, the small size of the cartilage and the inability to carve flanges limit its usefulness. The thyroid ala is exposed by dividing and retracting the strap muscles. The thyrohyoid muscles are dissected from the thyroid cartilage in a medial to lateral fashion, and a transverse incision is made through the cartilage 1–2 mm above the level of the vocal folds. Vertical incisions are made medially and laterally to allow for mobilization of the graft.

Auricular cartilage

Auricular cartilage can be useful in the management of suprastomal collapse as a cap graft or overlay graft. It is easily harvested but is relatively weak and may result in a cosmetic defect at the donor site, particularly in children <1 year of age.

Expansion procedures

Anterior cricoid split

The anterior cricoid split was developed in the 1980s as an alternative to performing a tracheotomy in infants who failed extubation (Cotton & Seid 1980). Patients had to meet strict criteria to be candidates for the procedure. As a result of advances in neonatal care, many of the infants who would have required an anterior cricoid split in the past are now managed without intubation, decreasing the need for this procedure. After exposing the larynx, an anterior laryngofissure extending through the lower one third of the thyroid cartilage is performed. The infant should remain intubated for 7–10 days postoperatively. Placing a thyroid ala graft increases the likelihood of success without adding significant operative morbidity (White et al. 2009). Additional modifications of the operation include splitting the posterior cricoid (open or endoscopically), endoscopic division of the anterior cricoid, or a combination of these procedures (Mirabile et al. 2010).

Laryngotracheal reconstruction (anterior costal cartilage graft)

Historically, double-stage laryngotracheal reconstruction (LTR) with anterior cartilage grafting was the cornerstone of subglottic stenosis (SGS) management. Currently, anterior graft LTR is used primarily to manage patients with failed endoscopic management, mild SGS (grade 1 or 2), or suprastomal collapse. Anterior graft LTR is typically performed as a single-stage procedure using thyroid ala or costal cartilage and has success rates >90% (Gustafson et al. 2000).

To perform an anterior graft LTR, the anterior airway is exposed from the thyroid notch to below the stenosis or below the stoma if a tracheostomy is present. The anterior cricoid cartilage is divided vertically in the midline extending the split superiorly or inferiorly as needed to span the entire length of the stenosis. The anterior commissure should not be violated. If necessary, endoscopic guidance may be used to complete the division; this is recommended in revision procedures to minimize risk to the vocal folds. In a single-stage LTR, the patient is intubated with an age-appropriate size endotracheal tube. In a double-stage procedure, a suprastomal stent may be placed. The appropriate length and width of the graft are determined, and the cartilage is carved into a boat-shape with flanges that prevent prolapse of the graft into the airway. The graft is secured using monofilament sutures using a mattress technique with the knots located laterally over the tracheal cartilage. A leak test is performed to ensure that the airway is sealed and fibrin glue may be placed judiciously around the anastomosis. If a thick layer of fibrin glue is placed covering the entire graft, the blood supply to the cartilage will be compromised. The strap muscles are closed over the graft to provide blood supply to the cartilage, and a Penrose drain is placed superficial to the strap muscles to avoid compromising the blood supply to the graft. In a single-stage procedure, the patient can be extubated from 0 to 7 days postoperatively.

In infants <9 months of age with symptomatic SGS, a single-stage anterior graft can be performed concomitantly with a posterior cricoid split. In these patients, the posterior cricoid split heals quickly enough to avoid the need for a posterior graft. Intubation for 7–10 days is usually sufficient to provide distraction of the posterior cricoid and to allow fibrosis to occur.

Laryngotracheal reconstruction (posterior costal cartilage graft)

A posterior cartilage graft LTR is indicated in patients with posterior glottic stenosis, high-grade SGS (grade 3 or 4), or bilateral vocal fold fixation due to paralysis or cricoarytenoid joint fixation. In some cases, a posterior graft is placed during laryngeal cleft repair. Costal cartilage is the most frequently used graft material. Patients with posterior glottic stenosis who have undergone posterior graft placement reportedly have an overall decannulation rate of 97% (Rutter & Cotton 2004).

The anterior cricoid cartilage is divided as described above. Ideally, the anterior commissure is preserved, which maintains the integrity of the thyroid cartilage and improves the stability of the larynx. If a complete laryngofissure is necessary, division of the anterior commissure should be performed under direct endoscopic visualization to minimize the risk of postoperative vocal dysfunction. The posterior cricoid lamina is then divided in the midline, and a round knife is used to create pockets on the posterior aspect of the cricoid plate to accommodate the flanges of the graft. The length of the desired graft is determined. To minimize the risk of postoperative aspiration, overdistraction of the posterior cricoid should be avoided. A 5 mm wide graft is sufficient in a 2-year-old and an 8–10 mm graft is adequate in a teenager. The graft is carved with a dorsal flange in a rectangular fashion, and is then 'snapped' into place, engaging the flanges under the cut edges of the posterior cricoid. In most cases, sutures are not required, but if the graft is unstable, sutures may be necessary. An age-appropriate endotracheal tube or suprastomal stent is placed to provide additional stabilization of the graft. The endotracheal tube is removed in 5–10 days, and the stent is left in place for 2–8 weeks. An anterior graft may be placed at this time if necessary.

Although commonly performed as an open procedure, a posterior graft may also be placed using an endoscopic approach. The patient is placed into suspension, and the posterior cricoid plate is divided endoscopically using cold instrumentation or a laser. The graft is then positioned endoscopically. As with the open procedure, this may be performed in a single- or double-stage fashion. A recent study demonstrated that 89% of patients who underwent endoscopic posterior graft placement were either successfully decannulated or avoided a tracheostomy (Gerber et al. 2013).

Laryngotracheal reconstruction (anterior and posterior grafts)

Anterior and posterior grafts are required in patients with high-grade SGS (grade 3 or 4), especially when a resection is contraindicated, and in patients in whom a resection has been previously performed. Reported success rates vary, ranging from 83% to 96% (Gustafson et al. 2000, Rutter & Cotton 2004, Smith et al. 2010).

Resection surgery

Cricotracheal resection

Cricotracheal resection (CTR) is an alternative to anterior and posterior cartilage LTR. The goal of a CTR is to remove the stenotic segment of the airway and reconnect the healthy superior and inferior segments. CTR is indicated in patients with severe SGS (grade 3 or 4) or a structurally inadequate subglottis and in patients who have undergone previous airway reconstruction. Relative contraindications to this procedure include low-grade SGS, stenosis within 3 mm of the vocal folds, or conditions that impair mobilization of the trachea such as previous distal tracheal surgery or previous injury to the tracheoesophageal septum. As with expansion procedures, CTR can be performed as a single- or double-stage procedure. Successful decannulation following CTR is achieved in >90% of patients.

At the beginning of the procedure, an esophageal bougie is placed to facilitate identification and avoidance of the esophagus. The anterior and lateral trachea is exposed from the thyroid cartilage to below the tracheostoma. Stay sutures are placed bilaterally to prevent retraction of the trachea into the chest. The proximal extent of the stenosis is identified using a 25-gauge needle under endoscopic guidance. The airway is then entered using either a vertical or horizontal incision. A vertical incision allows for conversion to a cartilage graft LTR if needed. A vertical incision has the advantage of preserving as many intact cartilage rings as possible. Regardless of whether the initial airway incision is vertical or horizontal, the goal is en bloc removal of the majority of the stenosis including the anterior cricoid and the anterior two thirds of the lateral cricoid. Care must be taken to avoid disruption of the cricothyroid joints, thereby minimizing risk to the recurrent laryngeal nerve.

After transection, the trachea is mobilized. The posterior cricoid mucosa is injected with lidocaine and incised at the upper border of the stenosis. The posterior cricoid plate is exposed, and the mucosa and scar tissue are dissected off the cricoid. The perichondrium is then incised again at the lower border of the cricoid cartilage, which leads directly into the plane between the trachea and the esophagus. The trachea is then mobilized off the esophagus posteriorly and exposed anteriorly to the level of the innominate artery. After ensuring that the proximal laryngeal and distal tracheal ends of the airway have adequate lumens, the anastomosis is started. Although the anastomosis has historically been performed using multiple interrupted sutures, we prefer to use a double-armed polydioxanone (PDS) suture starting posteriorly and working around both sides using a baseball suture until the lateral walls are reached. The patient is then nasotracheally intubated or a stent is placed and the lateral suture lines are carried up onto the anterior trachea until they meet in the midline. The stay sutures placed earlier in the procedure are then looped around the hyoid bone using a McGowan needle. Fibrin glue is placed over the anastomosis, and the wound is closed in layers over a Penrose drain. Chin-to-chest sutures may be placed between the mandibular and clavicular perichondrium. A cervical spine collar may be used instead of chin-to-chest sutures in older children and adults. In a single-stage procedure, the patient may be extubated immediately or on postoperative day 1. In younger children, several days of intubation are often required to allow for resolution of edema.

Tracheal resection

Tracheal resection with primary anastomosis is performed infrequently in children and has recently been supplanted by the cervical slide tracheoplasty.

Slide tracheoplasty

Originally developed as a procedure to repair congenital tracheal stenosis caused by complete tracheal rings, the slide tracheoplasty is presently used to repair stenosis due to absent tracheal rings, sleeve trachea, long-segment stenosis, 'A-frame' deformities, multilevel laryngotracheal anomalies, and select tracheoesophageal fistulae. Conceptually, the slide tracheoplasty overlaps the stenotic segments of the trachea, thereby shortening the trachea but doubling the circumference of the airway.

Intrathoracic slide tracheoplasty

A slide tracheoplasty may be performed using extracorporeal membrane oxygenation or jet ventilation. However, the use of cardiopulmonary bypass via a midline sternotomy facilitates the repair by eliminating the need for ventilation during the procedure and allowing for better exposure of the airway by decompressing the heart and lungs. Coexisting cardiovascular anomalies can be repaired through the same approach.

Once the patient is placed on cardiopulmonary bypass, the proximal and distal extents of the airway lesion are identified under direct endoscopic visualization using a 30-gauge needle. A beveled incision from proximal anterior to distal posterior is used to transect the airway at the midpoint of the stenosis. The proximal and distal segments of the trachea are mobilized by dissecting the soft tissue attachments between the posterior trachea and the esophagus. Lateral attachments should be preserved to protect the blood supply as well as the vagus and recurrent laryngeal nerves. The distal segment is split posteriorly, and the proximal segment is split anteriorly through the area of stenosis and into normal trachea. The edges of the split may be trimmed to facilitate closure. The anastomosis is performed in a posterodistal to anteroproximal fashion using a running continuous double-armed 4.0 PDS suture. Fibrin glue is placed along the anastomosis. The patient is taken off cardiopulmonary bypass, and the chest is closed. The airway is re-evaluated with a flexible bronchoscope to ensure that the repair is adequate and to clear blood and secretions from the airway. In the absence of cardiovascular comorbidities, the patient is extubated 24–48 hours following surgery.

In the largest cohort of patients to date (n = 80) who have undergone slide tracheoplasty on cardiopulmonary bypass, 63% were extubated within 48 hours of surgery and 30% required significant airway intervention (including multiple endoscopic procedures, stent placement, and revision surgery). The mortality in this cohort was only 5%, which is far lower than the reported mortality rate of 10–30% in patients with tracheal stenosis (Manning et al. 2011).

Cervical slide tracheoplasty

The cervical slide tracheoplasty is a modification of the intrathoracic slide tracheoplasty that provides a versatile alternative to the standard expansion and resection techniques (de Alarcon & Rutter 2012). The cervical approach avoids the need for cardiopulmonary bypass and is useful for pathology in the upper half to two thirds of the trachea. As in the intrathoracic slide tracheoplasty, the proximal and distal extents of the stenosis are identified under endoscopic visualization and the trachea is divided and split as described above. In patients with severe stenosis, partial resection may be performed. The anastomosis is performed using a double-armed PDS sutures as described above. In older children, the risk of developing a 'figure 8' deformity of the trachea is higher and a temporary silicone stent may be placed.

At the authors' institution, the cervical slide tracheoplasty has replaced tracheal resection in the management of upper tracheal stenosis, as it provides relative overexpansion of the trachea and the longer, oblique suture line minimizes the risk of anastomotic dehiscence and postoperative restenosis. In the largest study to date (n = 29) of patients who have undergone cervical slide tracheoplasty, 79% had operation-specific success and 90% experienced overall success (de Alarcon & Rutter 2012).

References

Cotton RT, Seid AB. Management of the extubation problem in the premature child: anterior cricoid split as an alternative to tracheotomy. Ann Otol Rhinol Laryngol 1980; 89:508–511.

de Alarcon A, Rutter MJ. Revision pediatric laryngotracheal reconstruction. Otolaryngol Clin North Am 2008; 41:959–980.

de Alarcon A, Rutter MJ. Cervical slide tracheoplasty. Arch Otolaryngol Head Neck Surg 2012; 138:812–816.

Gerber ME, Modi VK, Ward RF, Gower VM, Thomsen J. Endoscopic posterior cricoid split and costal cartilage graft placement in children. Otolaryngol Head Neck Surg 2013; 148:494–502.

Gustafson LM, Hartley BE, Liu JH, et al. Single-stage laryngotracheal reconstruction in children: a review of 200 cases. Otolaryngol Head Neck Surg 2000; 123:430–434.

Hartnick CJ, Hartley BE, Miller C, et al. Pediatric fiberoptic endoscopic evaluation of swallowing. Ann Otol Rhinol Laryngol 2000; 109:996–999.

Manning PB, Rutter MJ, Lisec A, Gupta R, Marino BS. One slide fits all: the versatility of slide tracheoplasty with cardiopulmonary bypass support for airway reconstruction in children. J Thorac Cardiovasc Surg 2011; 141:155–161.

McCormick ME, Johnson YJ, Pena M, et al. Dexmedetomidine as a primary sedative agent after single-stage airway reconstruction. Otolaryngol Head Neck Surg 2013; 148:503–508.

Meier JD, White DR. Multisystem disease and pediatric laryngotracheal reconstruction. Otolaryngol Clin North Am 2012; 45:643–651

Mirabile L, Serio P, Baggi R, Couloigner V. Endoscopic anterior cricoid split and balloon dilation in pediatric subglottic stenosis. Int J Pediatr Otorhinolaryngol 2010; 74:1409–1414.

Preciado D. Stenting in pediatric airway reconstruction. Laryngoscope 2012; 122:S97–S98.

Rutter MJ, Cotton RT. The use of posterior cricoid grafting in managing isolated posterior glottic stenosis in children. Arch Otolaryngol Head Neck Surg 2004; 130:737–739.

Simpson GT, Strong MS, Healy GB, et al. Predictive factors of success or failure in the endoscopic management of laryngeal and tracheal stenosis. Ann Otol Rhinol Laryngol 1982; 91:384–388.

Smith LP, Zur KB, Jacobs IN. Single- vs double-stage laryngotracheal reconstruction. Arch Otolaryngol Head Neck Surg 2010; 136:60–65.

Statham MM, de Alarcon A, Germann JN, et al. Screening and treatment of methicillin-resistant Staphylococcus aureus in children undergoing open airway surgery. Arch Otolaryngol Head Neck Surg 2012; 138:153–157.

White DR, Bravo M, Vijayasekaran S, et al. Laryngotracheoplasty as an alternative to tracheotomy in infants younger than 6 months. Arch Otolaryngol Head Neck Surg 2009; 135:445–447.

White DR, Cotton RT, Bean JA, et al. Pediatric cricotracheal resection: surgical outcomes and risk factor analysis. Arch Otolaryngol Head Neck Surg 2005; 131:896–899.

Willging JP. Benefit of feeding assessment before pediatric airway reconstruction. Laryngoscope 2000; 110:825–834.

12 Balloon dilation of the airway

Karthik Balakrishnan, Michael J Rutter

Historical overview

Airway dilation for the management of patients with laryngotracheal stenosis has been a mainstay of airway surgery for at least a century. For most of that period, dilation involved the passage of rigid or semirigid devices through the stenotic area. These devices included Jackson, cat-tail, and Maloney dilators, rigid bronchoscopes, and endotracheal tubes. All of these instruments produced inexorable shearing forces that damaged mucosa in both healthy and stenotic segments of the airway. Despite this considerable downside, dilation using a bougienage technique remained appealing, as it offered avoidance of external incisions, short operative time, and quick recovery.

The specific use of balloon catheters to widen stenotic segments of the airway was first reported by Cohen and colleagues in 1984 (Cohen et al. 1984). These authors described the use of angioplasty balloons to salvage the distal trachea and right mainstem bronchus of an infant with recurrent stenosis after excision of complete tracheal rings. Over the past several decades, balloon technology and techniques have expanded (Noppen et al. 1997, Lee et al. 2002, Mayse et al. 2004), becoming an invaluable tool for the management of airway stenosis. This chapter presents an overview of the advantages of this management approach, the types of balloons available, candidate and balloon selection, dilation techniques, adjunctive procedures, complications, and outcomes.

Advantages of balloon dilation

Case series published to date (Hebra et al. 1991, Lee & Rutter 2008, Whigham et al. 2012, Guarisco & Yang 2013), combined with our own clinical experience, suggest that balloons offer a number of advantages over other dilation instruments. First and most importantly, correctly placed balloons exert a purely radial expansile force on the stenotic area. Radial expansion also distributes force evenly over the circumference of the stenosis, thereby minimizing the risk of airway rupture at any single point.

Second, balloons permit the surgeon to fine-tune the force applied to the stenosis. Balloons expand through the instillation of fluid, using a device that incorporates a pressure gauge. This design allows ongoing fine adjustment of the pressure exerted by the balloon. In contrast, rigid dilators exert a radial force once they are in place; however, this force can be adjusted only by removing the dilator and inserting a larger one.

Each removal and insertion exerts shearing forces on the stenosis and potentially on the normal mucosa of the airway above and below the stenosis, as well as on the vocal folds. This shearing may cause injury and may cause edema and scarring as well as mucosal bleeding.

A third advantage of balloon dilation catheters is their shape and flexibility. Since these catheters were initially designed for use in angioplasty, they are long, narrow, and flexible – properties that are all beneficial in the airway. A narrow, flexible balloon may be steered through a severe stenosis, while the catheter's length allows the surgeon to reach more distal stenoses.

Indications for balloon dilation

Patient selection

Appropriate patient selection is crucial to the success of airway balloon dilation. In general, ideal candidates are patients with adequate cardiopulmonary reserve to allow airway occlusion or those with a tracheostomy and stenosis above the tracheostoma. Stenoses that are likely to respond well to balloon dilation are thin or weblike and soft, and consist of immature scar tissue. Firm or mature scar tissue, cartilaginous airway narrowing, and structural problems of the airway exoskeleton (e.g. complete rings, subglottic lateral shelves, A-frame deformity, and missing cartilage) are less likely to respond to dilation. In addition, dilation is less likely to achieve desired outcomes in longer stenoses; however, there is no maximum length beyond which dilation should not be attempted. Also noteworthy, in patients with second airway lesions, balloon dilation may be less likely to yield positive outcomes, as dilation of a single stenotic area may not provide an overall adequate airway (Whigham et al. 2012).

In general, balloon dilation requires the presence of an airway lumen large enough to permit entry of the deflated balloon. Stenoses with a pinpoint lumen may be gently dilated with a stylet and small cuffless endotracheal tubes until they are temporarily large enough for the surgeon to pass a balloon. Balloon dilation is therefore not generally suitable for the treatment of grade 4 stenosis.

Use as an adjunct to open airway reconstruction

Balloon dilation can be a useful adjunct to planned airway expansion or reconstruction procedures. In this context, the aim of dilation is to maintain patency of the airway lumen until the definitive procedure can be carried out. In patients with progressive grade 3 subglottic stenosis (>70% narrowing), interval balloon dilations may prevent the development of a complete (grade 4) stenosis that might preclude reconstruction with grafts (Guarisco & Yang 2013). Similarly, dilation may reduce the severity of a stenosis, permitting a single-stage procedure rather than a double-stage procedure. Dilations may be performed repeatedly until the patient is old enough or has sufficient growth to undergo open reconstruction.

Balloon dilation may also be used after airway reconstruction. Although postoperative dilation cannot be performed with a stent in place, once the stent is removed and adequate time is allowed for the reconstruction to heal, the balloon can be used in several ways. More specifically, in cases of postoperative edema or granulation, dilation may be combined with topical antibiotic/steroid drops to promote healing and reduce the risk of restenosis. Dilation may also be used to gently reposition an anterior graft that has prolapsed into the airway. Given that this particular use of the balloon carries the risk of displacing the graft, and that dilation after reconstruction generally has the potential to damage the repair, it should be done judiciously, at low pressures and with relatively small balloons.

Balloon selection

Balloon catheter design

All balloon catheters currently used for airway dilation have two ports (**Figure 12.1**). The first port is the inflation port, which allows the introduction of fluid to inflate the balloon. This port is usually labeled *balloon* (Boston Scientific, Natick, MA) or *B* (Acclarent, Inc, Menlo Park, CA) and is designed for attachment to the inflation device. The second port is used to introduce a stylet. Inadvertent instillation of inflation fluid through this port results in lung lavage rather than balloon inflation.

Semicompliant balloons

Although semicompliant balloons are not used at the authors' institution, these balloons are preferred by many surgeons. In contrast to noncompliant balloons, they are capable of expanding to different diameters at different pressures. When the portion of the balloon within the stenosis reaches an outward pressure equal to the

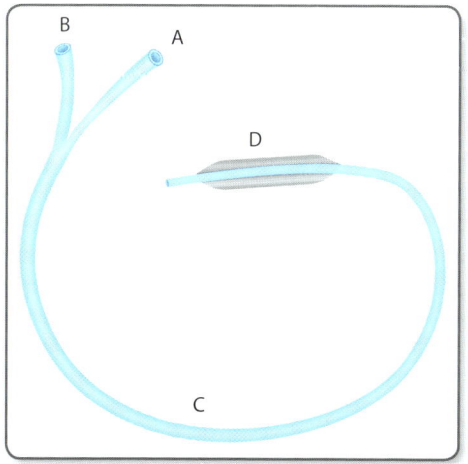

Figure 12.1 Basic schematic of an airway balloon catheter. Key components of the device are labeled. (A) Stylet port. (B) Inflation port. (C) Catheter shaft. (D) Balloon.

inward pressure exerted by the stenosis on the balloon, equilibrium is reached. As more fluid is introduced, the pressure at the stenosis and the balloon diameter at the stenosis remain relatively constant while the compliant balloon material allows the excess fluid to selectively fill the balloon above and below the stenosis. The result is an hourglass shape. Although these balloons have the advantage of exerting a constant pressure at the stenosis, they also have several important disadvantages. Most importantly, pressure equilibrium within the stenosis may be reached at a balloon diameter much smaller than the goal airway lumen diameter. In addition, the hourglass shape of the balloon may place excessive pressure on the mucosa above and below the stenosis, and these balloons cannot sustain as high a pressure at a given diameter as noncompliant balloons, as described subsequently.

Noncompliant balloons

Noncompliant balloons are designed to reach a uniform diameter over the full length of the balloon. This design allows the balloon to apply the greatest pressure and achieve full dilation at the narrowest point of the stenosis, thus avoiding the hourglass shape that may place undesirable pressure on adjacent areas of mucosa. These balloons may exert high pressures at the stenosis, making them more useful for dense scar tissue but raising the risk of airway rupture.

Balloon size and pressure selection

The surgeon's choice of balloon length and diameter is dependent upon the clinical context of the stenosis and the patient to be treated. In general, when using balloon dilation as a definitive treatment for airway stenosis from the glottis to the carina, the first step is to determine the diameter of an age-appropriate normal airway. For the subglottis and trachea, this is easily accomplished using endotracheal tube sizes, using the following equation:

Tube size = (age in years/4) + 4

Once the appropriate endotracheal tube size is selected, 1 mm is added to the outer diameter of that tube to determine the appropriate balloon diameter for use in the larynx. For tracheal dilation, the surgeon should add 2 mm rather than 1 mm. The difference between laryngeal and tracheal diameters reflects the anatomic difference between the closed ring of the cricoid and the open rings of the trachea. From the starting point established by these calculations, the surgeon can make adjustments, using smaller balloons for initial dilation of severe stenoses or relatively fresh reconstructions.

The target inflation pressure is usually determined by the 'burst pressure' of the balloon (i.e. the pressure beyond which the balloon may fail), which is specified on the packaging for each balloon. Generally, burst pressure becomes lower as balloon diameter becomes larger. Unless the surgeon has a specific reason to use a lower pressure, it is reasonable to use the burst pressure as the target inflation pressure.

Technique

Anesthesia

In patients without a tracheostomy, we prefer to perform endoscopy and dilation with the patient spontaneously ventilating. This technique requires close cooperation and good communication between the surgeon and the anesthesiologist. General anesthesia is typically induced with propofol and maintained with insufflated sevoflurane. If needed, the patient can temporarily be intubated above the stenotic area to allow maximal preoxygenation prior to dilation. Once the patient is adequately anesthetized, the surgeon should apply a weight-appropriate dose of topical laryngotracheal anesthetic. Prior to balloon insertion, the anesthesiologist should be informed that the airway will be fully occluded. In addition, the anesthesiologist should inform the surgeon when the oxyhemoglobin saturation drops to 90–92%, so that the balloon can be deflated and removed in a timely manner without excessive desaturation. The surgeon must be prepared to immediately provide mask ventilation once the balloon is removed in order to allow prompt reoxygenation. If the patient begins to 'cough' or 'buck' during balloon inflation, the balloon should be deflated and removed immediately and mask ventilation performed. Doing otherwise risks negative pressure pulmonary edema (NPPE) (as the patient attempts to inspire against the occluded airway), as well as barotrauma (when the patient forcefully exhales against the occluded airway). Once the patient is brought to a deeper level of anesthesia, dilation can be attempted again. The risk of NPPE is higher in adults and is rarely seen in children.

In patients with a tracheostomy and stenosis above the tracheostoma, airway management during dilation is much more straightforward. The tracheostomy tube may be left in place or replaced with a cuffed endotracheal tube through the stoma. The balloon can then be placed via direct laryngoscopy (described below) and inflated, while the anesthesiologist maintains oxygenation and ventilation via the tracheostoma. In this situation, the surgeon must ensure that the balloon does not ride under or next to the tracheostomy tube. Inflation with the balloon in such a position could force the tracheostomy tube against the tracheal wall and cause injury.

Dilation

The application of topical laryngotracheal anesthetic is strongly recommended, along with a diagnostic laryngoscopy and bronchoscopy immediately prior to dilation. This allows the surgeon to fully survey the airway and the stenotic area. Once this is done, the patient is preoxygenated and dilation can proceed. Under direct laryngoscopic visualization, the catheter is passed through the glottis to approximately the depth of the stenosis. The authors do not typically use a stylet, as the increased rigidity associated with the stylet raises the risk of airway perforation. The stylet may, however, be useful if a curve must be introduced into the catheter. If the catheter must be bent, it should be bent with the stylet in place to avoid kinking the inflation system.

With the assistant holding the balloon catheter in position, a narrow Hopkins Rod telescope is introduced and used to confirm that the balloon is centered within the stenosis. With the telescope still in place, the balloon is inflated to the target pressure. This telescopic visualization allows the surgeon to detect complications such as balloon failure or balloon displacement. Inflation is achieved using sterile saline. Water or air should not be used (**Figure 12.2**).

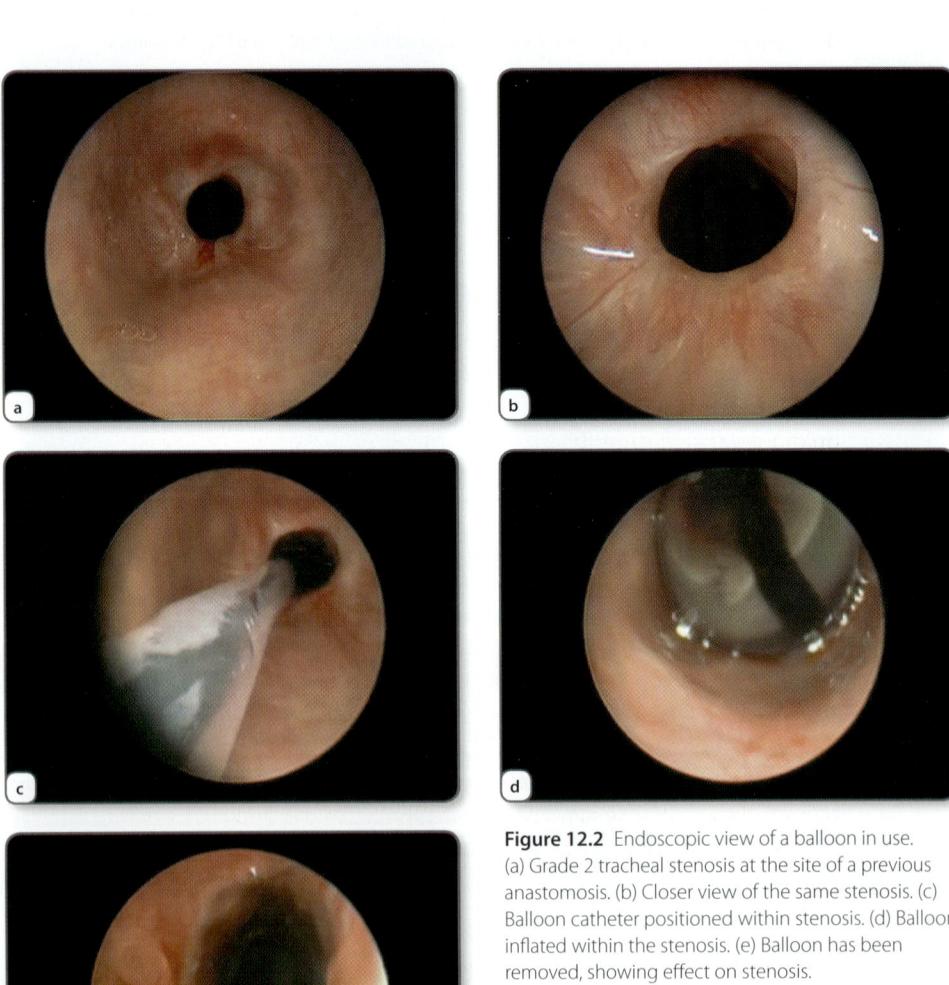

Figure 12.2 Endoscopic view of a balloon in use. (a) Grade 2 tracheal stenosis at the site of a previous anastomosis. (b) Closer view of the same stenosis. (c) Balloon catheter positioned within stenosis. (d) Balloon inflated within the stenosis. (e) Balloon has been removed, showing effect on stenosis.

After dilation is achieved, the balloon is completely deflated and removed. The telescope is left in place to visualize complete balloon deflation and to evaluate the dilated area for improved patency and for any complications such as tracheal injury.

Duration of dilation

The duration of dilations is ultimately limited by the inability to ventilate and oxygenate the patient while the balloon is inflated; within these limits, the optimal duration is unclear. Some surgeons prefer to use a fixed, arbitrary target time such as 2 minutes per dilation; however, data supporting this duration are lacking. An alternative method is to closely observe the pressure gauge on the balloon inflator. After the balloon is inflated to target pressure, the pressure will slowly drift downward as collagen crosslinks within the scar give way. The balloon can then be briefly inflated back to the target pressure for a total of 2 minutes and then deflated and removed.

Repeat dilation

Balloon dilation may be used repeatedly on the same lesion. In many cases, the initial dilation will achieve the full desired effect. Edema, granulation, and collapse may recur after dilation, and dilation itself may promote recurrent scarring. Accordingly, reassessment and patient and family education regarding the possibility of repeat dilation is essential.

The number of dilation attempts beyond which benefits plateau is unknown, and this number likely varies among patients. The timing of repeat dilation also varies widely. At the authors' institution, however, dilation is generally performed at 1- to 2-week intervals. If a patient does not show incremental benefit with a fourth dilation, other strategies are typically investigated, including open reconstruction. Regardless of the strategy chosen, the surgeon must evaluate the patient carefully at each dilation, comparing images and videos of previous endoscopic procedures.

Adjunctive procedures

Multiple procedures may be used to augment the effects of dilation. In general, these procedures are best performed with suspension microlaryngoscopy, which allows the surgeon to use a microscope or telescope to visualize the procedure, while leaving both hands free.

Scar division

In patients with thicker cicatricial scar tissue or stenoses that are not cartilaginous but are refractory to dilation alone, radial incisions can be made immediately prior to dilation. The authors typically make three radial incisions with a Blitzer knife or laser in what is often referred to as a 'Mercedes-Benz' configuration; one incision is made anteriorly and one is made posterolaterally on each side (**Figure 12.3**). These incisions create weak points in the scar, allowing dilation to produce controlled tears through the scar tissue. To reduce the risk of tearing

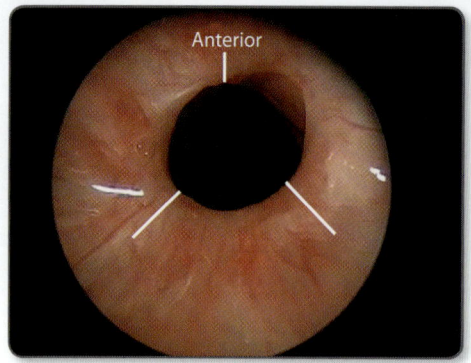

Anterior

Figure 12.3 Typical radial incisions made in a 'Mercedes-Benz' configuration, shown as white lines on this grade 2 stenosis. To reduce the risk of tearing into the trachealis muscle or creating a tracheoesophageal fistula, no direct posterior incision is made.

into the trachealis muscle or creating a tracheoesophageal fistula, no direct posterior incision is made.

Steroid injection

Steroid injection may be a useful addition in cases of refractory stenosis, particularly when underlying inflammatory process is suspected. This combination has been beneficial in treating patients with Wegener's granulomatosis (granulomatosis with polyangiitis) who have subglottic stenosis (Hoffman et al. 2003) and is being used with increasing frequency in children. The authors prefer the use of triamcinolone (40 mg/mL) via an orotracheal injection device under telescopic visualization. Injection is best given prior to dilation, as dilation flattens the stenosis, making injection more difficult. Injection prior to dilation may also be preferable because the pressure from the balloon may distribute the steroid throughout the scar.

Stenting

In cases of postreconstruction stenosis that is refractory to dilation alone, the combination of balloon dilation and stenting may be useful. Dilation is performed to achieve an age-appropriate airway lumen. Immediately following, a cut T-tube or Hood stent is placed endoscopically in patients without a tracheostoma, whereas a suprastomal stent or T-tube is placed in patients with a tracheostoma (Guarisco & Yang 2013).

Fluoroscopy

Historically, the use of balloon dilation catheters in the airway often involved fluoroscopy to confirm balloon placement. With the refinement of endoscopic balloon dilation techniques, this measure is no longer necessary for lesions of the larynx and trachea, as it not only carries the risks of radiation in pediatric patients but is also associated with additional costs, equipment, and staffing needs. Although fluoroscopy remains in use for lesions of the bronchi and more distal airways, continuous improvements in flexible bronchoscopic technology have made it comparatively less desirable.

Balloons via flexible bronchoscopes

Although lesions as distal as the mainstem bronchi are easily visualized with rigid telescopes, more distal stenoses and stenoses in patients with difficult airway access are better reached with flexible bronchoscopes. Flexible bronchoscopes currently provide excellent image quality and a working channel that allows the passage of a balloon catheter or other flexible instruments. Before passing the flexible bronchoscope into the airway, the surgeon should ensure that the working channel is wide enough to pass the catheter easily. For reference, 2.8- and 3.5 mm flexible bronchoscopes provide a 1.2 mm working channel, and 4.9 mm flexible bronchoscopes provide a 2.0 mm working channel. The latter is usually adequate to pass a balloon catheter. The balloon catheter must also be sufficiently long to pass entirely through the working channel, as inflation with the balloon partially within the channel may damage the bronchoscope. When dilating the bronchi, the surgeon should choose a balloon with a diameter equal to the normal airway lumen rather than upsizing by 1–2 mm, as is done for the larynx and trachea. Consideration may be given to the use of a guidewire to facilitate balloon placement through the working channel and stenosis; however, this may increase the risk of perforation.

Complications

Negative pressure pulmonary edema

As discussed earlier in this chapter, respiratory effort against an occluded airway may result in NPPE. In the case of balloon dilation, this complication is most likely to occur with attempted inspiration while the balloon is dilated. However, NPPE may also occur in patients with severe stenosis after dilation is completed and the balloon removed. In patients with a tracheostoma and stenosis above the stoma, this complication is rarely seen, as the stoma prevents development of significant negative pressure.

The cardinal sign of this complication is the production of copious, frothy, pinkish secretions from the airway. Lung compliance is reduced, and oxygenation and ventilation are compromised. Management includes immediately deflating and removing the balloon and providing positive-pressure ventilation. Subsequent management is medical. The patient should be transported to an intensive care setting, mechanical ventilation instituted, and consideration given to diuretics, morphine, nitrates, and supplemental oxygen therapy.

Airway rupture

Mechanical injury to the airway from balloon dilation may include mucosal abrasions and lacerations as well as full-thickness rupture. Perforation may result from direct trauma from the tip of the balloon catheter during catheter placement or from radial force exerted during dilation. Direct trauma can be avoided by placing the balloon under laryngoscopic or telescopic visualization and not advancing it blindly if resistance is met. Rupture can be avoided through appropriate selection of balloon type, diameter, and inflation pressure.

Small ruptures may be asymptomatic and go undetected, whereas more significant ruptures perforations may become evident with the use of positive-pressure ventilation. Signs and symptoms may include dyspnea, crepitus, or subcutaneous air; diminished lung sounds in the case of associated pneumothorax; or hypotension and tachycardia with a large pneumothorax or pneumomediastinum. Posterior perforations may also result in tracheoesophageal or bronchoesophageal fistulae. Management includes endotracheal intubation beyond the level of the perforation, return to spontaneous (negative-pressure) ventilation as soon as possible, serial imaging, and placement of a chest tube if needed. A nasogastric tube may be useful in cases of tracheoesophageal fistula, although placement should be done under endoscopic visualization to avoid propagating the fistula. In many patients, nonoperative management is sufficient to allow healing of the perforation. However, in patients with more severe injuries or injuries that do not heal spontaneously, operative repair may be necessary.

Airway obstruction

Airway obstruction may result from post-dilation edema, a clot in the airway from dilation-related bleeding, or from actual detachment or fracture of the balloon catheter with retention of the balloon in the airway. In the setting of edema, if positive pressure cannot achieve ventilation, prompt introduction of a small endotracheal tube or rigid bronchoscope may be lifesaving. In the setting of a clot in the airway, suctioning with or without saline lavage may be useful. For a retained balloon, the surgeon should puncture the balloon with a sharp instrument and then withdraw the balloon using an endoscopic grasper. If the balloon is high in the airway, a large-bore needle may also be used to transcutaneously puncture and deflate the balloon.

Balloon displacement ('watermelon seeding')

If the balloon is not centered within the stenosis prior to inflation, it will tend to slide proximally or distally as it is inflated. This problem is more likely to occur with noncompliant balloons and balloons that have a large diameter. It is particularly apparent when the rounded 'shoulders' at the ends of the balloon are within the stenotic segment. The surgeon must resist the temptation to put traction or pressure on the catheter to hold it in place, as this maneuver may kink the catheter and impede balloon deflation. Rather, the balloon should be fully deflated, repositioned, and reinflated once it is centered on the narrowest portion of the stenosis. Nonslip balloons currently under development may reduce or obviate this problem.

Inadvertent airway lavage

Inadvertent introduction of inflation fluid through the noninflation port will result in the escape of that fluid from the distal end of the catheter, filling the lower airways. The same complication may occur if the balloon fails, releasing fluid into the airway. Inadvertent airway lavage is easily recognized by the introduction of inflation fluid with no resulting inflation of the balloon or rupture of the balloon. Both possibilities can easily be detected by using a telescope to visualize the balloon during inflation. Management includes removal of the balloon catheter and suctioning of the trachea and lower airways to clear the fluid. Dilation can usually be attempted after suctioning is completed.

Balloon failure

For the most part, balloon failure can be avoided by taking care not to inflate the balloon beyond its specified burst pressure. Placing the end of the illuminated telescope close to the balloon during endoscopy may result in heat transfer to the balloon, with weakening and failure of the balloon wall. Balloon failure may be recognized by a sudden loss of pressure on the inflation gauge or rapid deflation visible under the telescope. As described above, balloon failure may result in airway lavage, requiring suctioning and another attempt at dilation with a fresh balloon. In this clinical scenario, consideration should be given to using a larger balloon to allow dilation to a larger diameter at lower pressure. Unlike endotracheal tube or tracheostomy tube cuffs, balloon catheters should not be tested by inflation prior to insertion, as their shape may change when deflated again, making insertion difficult.

Conclusion

Balloon dilation is an invaluable tool for managing airway stenosis in children. Whether used adjunctively or as the sole approach to maintaining or improving airway patency, it enables the airway surgeon to endoscopically manage a wide spectrum of laryngotracheal lesions. Sequential dilations can be performed, and these do not preclude later open reconstructive procedures. Dilation may also be used as a bridge to open reconstruction in appropriately selected cases. It is important to note that it can influence endoluminal scarring but is not as effective for problems of the laryngotracheal exoskeleton. The overall success of this approach therefore rests on careful patient selection and the use of balloons that are appropriate in regard to both size and design.

Acknowledgment

The authors would like to thank Aliza P Cohen for her assistance in writing this chapter.

References

Cohen MD, Weber TR, Rao CC. Balloon dilatation of tracheal and bronchial stenosis. Am J Roentgenol 1984; 142:477–478.

Guarisco JL, Yang CJ. Balloon dilation in the management of severe airway stenosis in children and adolescents. J Pediatr Surg 2013; 48:1676–1681.

Hebra A, Powell D, Smith CD, Othersen HB, Jr. Balloon tracheoplasty in children: results of a 15-year experience. J Pediatri Surg 1991; 26:957–961.

Hoffman GS, Thomas-Golbanov CK, Chan J, Akst LM, Eliachar I. Treatment of subglottic stenosis, due to Wegener's granulomatosis, with intralesional corticosteroids and dilation. J Rheumatol 2003; 30:1017–1021.

Lee KH, Ko GY, Song HY, Shim TS, Kim WS. Benign tracheobronchial stenoses: long-term clinical experience with balloon dilation. J Vasc Interv Radiol 2002; 13:909–914.

Lee KH, Rutter MJ. Role of balloon dilation in the management of adult idiopathic subglottic stenosis. Ann Otol Rhinol Laryngol 2008; 117:81–84.

Mayse ML, Greenheck J, Friedman M, Kovitz KL. Successful bronchoscopic balloon dilation of nonmalignant tracheobronchial obstruction without fluoroscopy. Chest 2004; 126:634–637.

Noppen M, Schlesser M, Meysman M, et al. Bronchoscopic balloon dilatation in the combined management of postintubation stenosis of the trachea in adults. Chest 1997; 112:1136–1140.

Whigham AS, Howell R, Choi S, et al. Outcomes of balloon dilation in pediatric subglottic stenosis. Ann Otol Rhinol Laryngol 2012; 121:442–448.

13 | Surgical management of the oncologic airway

Sandeep Samant, Jonathan P Giurintano

Introduction

Tumors arising from the mucosal surfaces and soft tissues of the head and neck often contribute to airway compromise either at the time of presentation or during or after the course of treatment. Management of actual or potential compromise of the airway due to head and neck tumors requires consideration of multiple factors, including tumor location, behavior, growth rate, and the designated multimodality treatment plan in addition to the patient-specific factors of anatomy, comorbidity, and functional status. Intervention throughout the course of managing these patients, from diagnosis to post-treatment surveillance, can have implications on the long-term health, quality of life, and even the likelihood of survival. Hence, such patients are most effectively managed under the supervision of expert physicians who routinely care for patients with head and neck tumors.

Clinical assessment

History and physical examination

Patients with tumors of the head and neck may initially present on an outpatient or emergent basis, with or without symptoms of airway compromise. Clinical evaluation must include a detailed history, thorough physical examination of the head and neck, biopsy to ascertain pathological diagnosis, and imaging to delineate the anatomic extent of involvement as well as, if necessary, to assess the extent of airway compromise.

Initial evaluation of the patient should determine whether airway compromise is acutely imminent. The presence of stridor or severe stertor, the use of accessory muscles for respiration, and an anxious appearance or feeling of impending doom suggest severe obstruction of the airway that requires urgent attention. Several important clues can be obtained upon initial observation of a patient in respiratory distress. A patient with an obstructive oropharyngeal mass may be unable to lie supine without struggling to breathe, forcing the patient to sit up and lean forward to breathe comfortably. Obstruction at the supraglottis or glottis presents with audible inspiratory stridor, while a mass located in the subglottis or trachea may present with biphasic stridor and prolongation of the inspiratory and expiratory phases of respiration.

If the patient is in no acute distress, attention should be focused on obtaining a detailed history and physical examination. Two presenting complaints frequently seen in head and neck cancer may imply impending airway compromise: voice change and dysphagia. A voice characterized by the patient as 'hoarse' suggests laryngeal involvement by tumor, whereas tumors of the oropharynx can produce a 'hot-potato' voice, and tumors of the nasopharynx may obstruct the velopharyngeal airway, yielding a hyponasal voice. Examination of the nasal and oral cavities, nasopharynx, oropharynx, hypopharynx, and larynx, ideally with flexible fiberoptic endoscopy, will quickly identify the location of obstructing tumor and help determine the patency of the remaining airway.

In the patient with head and neck cancer who is receiving or has completed surgical or adjuvant therapy, the exact treatment details should be elucidated. The presence of scars across the cervical neck, a 'woody' feeling upon palpation of the neck, or diffuse skin changes should alert the physician to a history of prior intervention for head and neck cancer. Previous surgical intervention may yield distortion of the normal airway anatomy, and radiation therapy to the neck and pharyngeal musculature can fibrose the soft tissues of the neck, resulting in trismus or limitation of forward displacement of the mandible upon retraction. Radiation therapy may also produce significant edema or necrosis of the laryngeal structures, narrowing the patency of the laryngeal inlet, distorting the shape of the epiglottis and aryepiglottic folds, and limiting vocal cord abduction. In this patient demographic, a history of prior surgery or radiation to the neck should always alert the physician about the potentially difficult nature of securing the patient's airway with standard measures, and there should be a lower threshold for pursuing a surgical airway.

Finally, the presence of any comorbidities should be elucidated, as reduction in the patient's cardiopulmonary reserve may affect choices that are made with regard to the clinical interventions for securing the airway.

Imaging

Computed tomography (CT) of the neck with and without contrast enhancement is the most useful imaging modality for patients with tumors affecting the head and neck, providing details essential for optimizing airway management along with the information necessary for clinically staging and treating the neoplasm. Information provided by CT includes the tumor's size, extent, and relation to vital anatomic structures such as the viscera, great vessels, nerves, bony facial skeleton, and the deep spaces of the neck. Mutiplanar reconstruction of the CT scan dataset is frequently valuable in making these assessments. Specifically, sagittal and coronal reconstructions can prove beneficial in assessing the patency of the laryngeal and tracheal airways. Volume rendering techniques that can demonstrate the three-dimensional relationship of the tumor to its surrounding structures and virtual endoscopy algorithms that can delineate regions of airway narrowing are also helpful for operative planning in select cases.

Magnetic resonance imaging (MRI) is of value in assessing the soft tissue extent of tumors, providing information regarding tumor vascularity, dural invasion, perineural extension, tumor spread along tissue planes beyond the primary tumor mass, and separation of tumor from secretions within sinus cavities. MRI is also useful in assessing the extent of tumor mass in lesions that occupy the lower neck and upper mediastinum, allowing the physician to study the relationship of these masses to the surrounding major blood vessels.

Ultrasonography (US) is most often used for imaging the thyroid, submandibular, and parotid glands. For the thyroid gland, US provides excellent structural detail within thyroid gland parenchyma, allowing determination of size and consistency of thyroid nodules or masses, presence of calcifications, and state of blood flow within and around the nodules. Additionally, US helps identify lymphadenopathy in the central compartment (level VI) and other nodal levels of the neck. Though US can display displacement or compression of the tracheal air column by a thyroid mass, it is inferior to CT in providing information regarding the extent of airway compromise or tracheal or laryngeal cartilage invasion. While US avoids the use of intravenous contrast and may be of benefit in patients with thyroid carcinoma who will later require treatment with radioactive iodine, when significant compromise of the airway is suspected, CT is the preferred imaging modality in order to plan safe surgical intervention.

Airway management considerations

Laryngeal cancer

Of all the locations of cancer in the head and neck, cancer of the larynx most often presents with symptoms of airway obstruction. Based on the anatomy of the laryngeal framework, laryngeal can be divided into three categories, each with its own distinct clinical behavior: supraglottic, glottic, and subglottic. Supraglottic tumors tend to present with dysphagia, odynophagia, and frequently obstruction of the supraglottic airway. Metastasis to the cervical lymph nodes is common and tends to be bilateral. Tumors arising from the glottis tend to present at an earlier stage than supraglottic tumors, as the presentation of persistent hoarseness warrants earlier referral to an otolaryngologist, and the glottis larynx contains structural barriers to tumor spread. However, if glottis tumors persist, they may cause mechanical obstruction of the glottis airway as well as fixation of the vocal cords, resulting in airway compromise. The most rare laryngeal cancer, subglottic tumors tend to portend a poor prognosis and are commonly associated with tumor spread inferiorly into the trachea, late presentation, and lymphatic metastasis to the central compartment of the neck and upper mediastinum by the time of diagnosis (**Figure 13.1**).

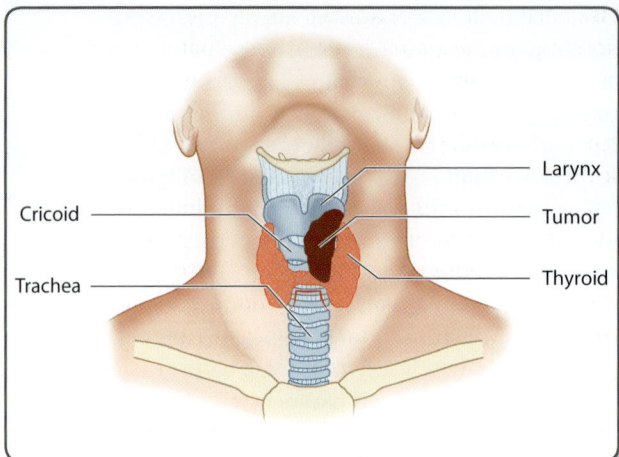

Figure 13.1 Lymphatic metastasis of tumor to the central compartment of the neck, with key anatomic landmarks highlighted.

Larynx

Cricoid

Tumor

Trachea

Thyroid

If a patient with laryngeal cancer presents with audible stridor, an anxious appearance, and use of accessory muscles for respiration, the safest airway intervention is generally to proceed to the operating room for an awake tracheotomy performed under local anesthesia. If the patient is not acutely decompensating, flexible fiberoptic laryngoscopy will reveal the location of the tumor, presence of any bleeding, and movement of the vocal cords, and also allow the surgeon to determine whether orotracheal intubation is feasible. Obtaining a CT of the neck with and without contrast prior to proceeding to the operating room is preferred if the patient is stable. This imaging will help delineate the extent of the lesion. From a surgical standpoint, it is important to study the most inferior extent of the tumor to avoid entering the trachea in an area involved by tumor, as tracheotomy at the location of tumor will result in contamination of the tracheotomy site with malignant cells, greatly increasing the probability of subsequent tracheostomal cancer recurrence.

In the operating room, patient should be placed supine on the operating table with a shoulder roll to place the neck into extension, providing optimal visualization of the trachea. If the patient is unable to lie supine without becoming dyspneic, the head of bed may be elevated until the patient is in a more comfortable position. Continuous supplemental oxygen is delivered via nasal cannula; a minimal amount of monitored sedation and anxiolytic may be used to relax the patient without causing respiratory depression.

The cricoid cartilage is palpated, and the skin and soft tissue inferior to the cricoid are generously anesthetized with 1% lidocaine with 1:100,000 epinephrine to provide sufficient local anesthesia. A limited vertical incision is made in the midline immediately inferior to the cricoid. It is of utmost importance not to extend this incision too far superiorly, as this may compromise the incision for a future total laryngectomy. If there is concern for inadequate access via this limited vertical incision due to surgeon inexperience or patient anatomy, a horizontal incision placed 1 cm below the inferior border of the cricoid cartilage may be used as well.

The most critical step in performing tracheotomy on a patient with laryngeal cancer is correct placement of the initial tracheal entry and subsequent tracheal flap. Attention must be paid to determining the inferior limit of the laryngeal tumor in order to prevent entry into the larynx at the site of tumor. While preparing for a possible future total laryngectomy, tracheal entry should be placed as superior as possible without exposing tumor so that there is maximum length of cervical trachea that can be used for creation of a healthy tracheostoma. A horizontal incision through the interspace between the first and second or the second and third tracheal rings is ideal. The author prefers a limited inferiorly based Bjork flap extending no more than a single tracheal ring to allow for the tracheotomy tube to be comfortably introduced without any posterior buckling of the anterior tracheal wall. A flap longer than this will compromise the length of trachea available for creating a healthy tracheostoma should the patient need a total laryngectomy.

If the patient is not in severe enough distress to warrant urgent awake tracheostomy, one must determine whether a tracheotomy can be avoided altogether prior to commencing therapy. Intravenous corticosteroids can reduce inflammatory edema of the soft tissue surrounding the tumor, often sufficiently relieving the mechanical obstruction to allow commencement of therapy, obviating the need for tracheotomy. If a pathologic diagnosis of the tumor has not been made and direct laryngoscopy must be performed for obtaining a tissue sample, the decision should be made as to whether the patient can be safely intubated. If flexible fiberoptic laryngoscopy demonstrates presence of an airway, an awake fiberoptic nasal intubation may be performed to help guide the endotracheal tube past the tumor into the tracheal lumen. Alternatively, an 'awake-look' using a standard or videoscopic rigid laryngoscope can be undertaken after adequately anesthetizing the oropharynx and laryngeal inlet with a topical anesthetic. A superior laryngeal nerve block may be performed to anesthetize the supraglottic larynx if felt necessary. It is prudent to maintain spontaneous ventilation in case the airway is unable to be secured with these techniques; as such, paralytic agents must be used with extreme caution.

Intubating the patient with laryngeal cancer can be risky, as there is the possibility of losing the airway due to laryngospasm or bleeding from an exophytic tumor. The importance of open and detailed communication between the surgeon and anesthesiologist cannot be overstated. Because of the possibility of unsuccessful intubation, a tracheostomy tray with a 15-blade scalpel and several tracheostomy tubes should be opened and ready for use in case an emergency tracheotomy is necessary.

Once the patient has been intubated, the surgeon must determine whether debulking the tumor can improve the airway patency and avoid a tracheotomy. Although there is some controversy regarding the utility of tumor debulking in the literature, there is a preponderance of evidence that suggests tracheotomy may increase the likelihood of stomal recurrence after total laryngectomy. In the process of tumor debulking, care must be taken not to disrupt vital laryngeal structures such as the vocal cords or arytenoids even if they are involved by tumor, as they may recover function after radiation therapy. If the surgeon feels confident that the patient will tolerate extubation, a tracheotomy may be avoided. It is vital that the patient is watched closely in the operating room after extubation to ensure that the airway is satisfactory and stable.

In carefully selected patients with partial obstruction, initial treatment with a cycle of induction chemotherapy [e.g. TPF (cisplatin, paclitaxel, and 5-fluorouracil)] may be administered under observation in the hospital in order to shrink tumor volume reduction so as to avoid tracheotomy.

All measures mentioned above require significant familiarity with the treatment of head and neck cancer and must never be undertaken at any significant risk of loss of airway. In the absence of adequate anesthesia, surgical equipment, or facilities for adequate monitoring and prompt intervention if needed, it is always safer to perform a tracheotomy.

Hypopharyngeal cancer

Cancer of the hypopharynx arises most commonly in the pyriform sinuses. Other locations of origin include posterior hypopharyngeal wall and the postcricoid area. Pyriform sinus and postcricoid tumors may quickly invade the larynx, causing airway obstruction by a combination of tissue edema in the paraglottic space, tumor extension into the supraglottic larynx, and recurrent laryngeal nerve paralysis. Considerations for management of such patients are identical to those discussed for laryngeal cancer in the preceding section.

Oropharyngeal tumors

Tumors of the oropharynx (tonsil, base of tongue, soft palate, or posterior pharyngeal wall) only present with airway obstruction in the late stages but may difficult to manage if they are bulky and occupy the oropharyngeal airspace. As oropharyngeal tumors are often exophytic and may easily hemorrhage with manipulation, administration of paralytic agents should be avoided until laryngeal inlet has been visualized. Flexible fiberoptic-guided intubation may be used as an option, but precaution must be taken against inducing bleeding during intubation attempts. If intubation is unsuccessful or deemed to be too risky, a tracheotomy may become necessary. Tracheotomy should only be performed if general anesthesia is required for a biopsy to make a tissue diagnosis, and the patient may have continued airway compromise postoperatively.

Surgical intervention for tumors of the oropharynx may be performed either through the transoral route or through a more invasive approach such as a mandibular swing. Transoral resection with the help of a surgical robot (TORS) has become increasingly utilized. TORS generally does not result in significant airway compromise in the postoperative period, and prophylactic preoperative tracheotomy is generally not necessary. However, more extensive surgery of the oropharynx requiring an open approach such as a mandibular swing always requires a temporary tracheotomy, especially if a microvascular or regional flap is performed concurrently. Once sufficient time has passed to allow decrease in edema at the surgical site, decannulation may be considered.

Oral cavity tumors

Oral cavity tumors generally do not cause airway obstruction unless they are very advanced and extended into the oropharyngeal or laryngeal airways. If considerable disruption of the floor of mouth or tongue is required to obtain clear surgical margins, microvascular free tissue transfer may be necessary, in which case a tracheostomy is necessary.

Conclusion

Malignant tumors of head and neck often contribute to airway compromise and are ideally managed by surgeons who care for patients with head and neck cancer on a regular basis. Tumors of the oral cavity, oropharynx, nasopharynx, supraglottic larynx, glottic larynx, or subglottic larynx may all result in airway obstruction, though laryngeal tumors most often present with airway symptoms. If a patient with known or suspected head and neck cancer presents with airway distress, the physician must obtain a detailed clinical history including any prior history of radiation therapy, and CT imaging of the neck should be performed. The initial determination must be made: does the patient require emergent awake tracheotomy or not? If tracheotomy is not warranted, then the determination should be made: should the patient be intubated and tumor debulking performed, or could administration of intravenous corticosteroids or induction chemotherapy avoid a trip to the operating room? Regardless of the treatment modality pursued, it should always be kept in mind that patients with head and neck cancers may have tenuous airways before, during, and after cancer treatments, and a low threshold for medical or surgical intervention should be maintained for patients with head and neck cancer presenting with obstructive airway symptoms.

Further reading

Bradley PJ. Treatment of the patient with upper airway obstruction caused by cancer of the larynx. Otolaryngol Head Neck Surg 1999; 120:737–741.

Dougherty TB, Clayman GL. Airway management of surgical patients with head and neck malignancies. Anesth Clin North Am 1998; 16:547–562.

Dougherty TB, Nguyen DT. Anesthetic management of the patient scheduled for head and neck cancer surgery. J Clin Anesth 1994; 6:74–82.

Garg R, Darlong V, Pandey R, Punj J. Anesthesia for oncological ENT surgeries: review. Internet J Anesthesiol 2008; 20:1–7.

Jensen NF, Benumof JL. The difficult airway in head and neck tumour surgery. Anesth Clin North Am 1993; 11:475–511.

Londy F, Norton ML. Radiologic techniques for evaluation and management of the difficult airway. In: Norton ML, Brown ACD (eds), Atlas of the difficult airway. St. Louis: Mosby-Year Book, 1991:62.

Supkis DE Jr, Dougherty TB, Nguyen DT, Cagle CK. Anesthetic management of the patient undergoing head and neck cancer surgery. Int Anesthesiol Clin 1998; 36:21–29.

Supkis DE Jr. Anesthesia for the cancer patient: an overview. Anesth Clin North Am 1998; 16:511–532.

14

Difficult airway management in the complex patient

Francisco Vieira, Jared J Tompkins

Introduction

Management of the difficult airway remains one of the most challenging tasks for health-care service providers and practitioners. The initial step in an airway procedure is a thorough evaluation by the surgeon to anticipate and characterize the nature and grade of the airway. It takes time for a detailed airway examination, however, and it is not always possible in an acute emergency situation. Difficult airway complications in a hospital setting occur more frequently in the critical care setting (intensive care unit), followed by the emergency department, then the operating room during anesthesia.

Current evidence suggests that a great majority of events can be avoided with better airway assessment and management practices, including better utilization of awake intubation and knowledge of the appropriate use of supraglottic airway devices. A great number of adverse events can be attributed to judgment and training.

Knowledge of existing comorbidities in patients on long-term ventilator support is critical. One must weigh the benefit from the procedure against the unbiased implicated risks. These risks increase with anatomical confounders such as obesity, cancer, head and neck trauma, and a short neck with limited or decreased range of motion. These factors, when not taken seriously, may increase the odds of an unexpected outcome.

Of note, it is necessary to understand that successful intubation does not always result in successful ventilation. Objective measures such as a blood oxygen saturation >96% (measured by pulse oximetry), an absence of epigastric sounds, the presence of chest auscultation, bilateral excursion, endotracheal tube misting, or fiberoptic-assisted intubation are reassuring, but do not confirm ventilation. End-tidal CO_2 levels on capnography ultimately provide confirmation.

The difficult airway

A common definition of the difficult airway is the clinical situation in which a trained practitioner experiences difficulty with endotracheal intubation and/or difficulty with ventilation of the airway. Securing an airway urgently can pose a real technical challenge, even under favorable conditions. However, it can develop into an extreme challenge when presenting with substantial unfavorable factors, such as uncompensated diabetes mellitus, coagulopathies, obstructive sleep apnea (OSA), and cardiopulmonary diseases.

Management of the difficult airway depends mainly on the interrelation of three complex factors (**Figure 14.1**):

1. Patient status
2. Clinical setting
3. Skills of the practitioner

If more than one factor has been compromised, the result is a difficult or failed airway (Apfelbaum et al. 2013).

Predictors of a difficult airway

These include:

- Obesity: Short neck, false trajectory
- Trauma to the head and neck region, including spine fracture, trismus, maxillofacial instability, foreign body, or active bleeding
- Malignancy: upper aerodigestive tract cancer with airway obstruction, or previously irradiated neck
- Iatrogenic, for example infrastomal subglottic stenosis from previous tracheostomy mechanical trauma at a level below the sternum notch or a higher position of the carina associated with a high-lying innominate artery and pleural wall exposure due to emphysema, previous lung surgery, chest trauma, obesity, or pregnancy
- Idiopathic, for example tracheomalacia (can be asymptomatic) progressing under mechanical stress as a result of long-term intubation or overlapping infection
- Endocrine: thyroid goiter, coexistent hyperthyroidism, pregnancy.
- Degenerative diseases: Ankylosis, osteoarthritis risk of cervical subluxation
- Congenital: Down syndrome and other craniofacial anomalies

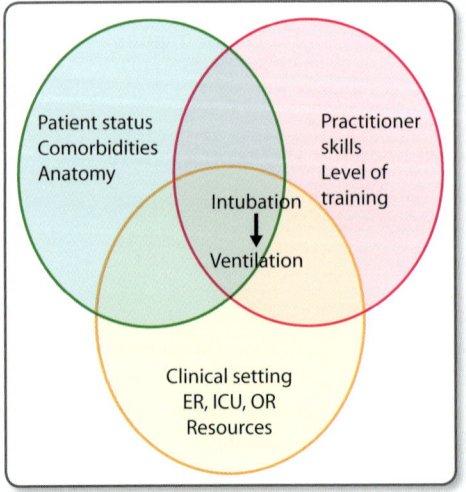

Figure 14.1 Patient status, clinical setting, and skills of the practitioner. All three factors need to be present, interacting in combination with each other.

Principal adverse events associated with the difficult airway

- Esophageal intubation
- Mainstem bronchial intubation
- Oxygen desaturation
- Pneumothorax
- Hypotension
- Aspiration
- Laryngospasm
- Cardiac arrhythmia
- Traumatic damage to the teeth
- Airway trauma
- Unnecessary surgical airway
- Anoxic brain injury
- Cardiopulmonary arrest
- Death

The complex patient and pre-existent medical comorbidities

There is no agreement among authors as to a precise definition of the complex patient, and there is no consensus on a quantitative definition relating the number of associated comorbidities needed to establish this designation. A qualitative definition has been discussed and defined as 'a patient with preceding illnesses in addition to the primary condition, requiring care beyond standard medical treatment' (Weiss 2007).

Several comorbidity indices exist, including the Charlson, Elixhauser, Kaplan–Feinstein, Higashi, and others. Intensive care unit, operating room, and emergency department practitioners utilize these predictive models, which assign a numerical value to comorbidities in order to quantify complexity (Charlson et al. 1987, Elixhauser et al. 1998, Higashi et al. 2007). These tools predict mortality risks after tracheotomy in terms of the coexisting conditions. Those patients with a higher comorbidity index showed a clear trend toward an increased rate of mortality (Meacham & Vieira 2012).

Medical conditions commonly requiring evaluation for tracheostomy in the ICU

These include:

- To assist weaning from ventilatory support in patients on intensive care
- Multisystem organ failure: liver, renal, pulmonary and failure
- Cardiac insufficiency: decompensated congestive heart failure, myocardial infarction
- Diabetes mellitus associated to obesity
- Respiratory failure: uncompensated COPD (if >50 years old and 20 pack/year smoker), acute pulmonary edema, pneumonia, pulmonary embolism, acute respiratory distress syndrome
- Neurologic disorders: cerebral vascular accident, coma, degenerative disorders

- HIV/AIDS, and other immunosuppressive disorders
- Cancer: locally advanced, metastatic extension
- Trauma: cervical spine injury, cranial trauma.
- Postsurgical complications
- Sepsis and other complicated infections
- Degenerative or connective tissue disease
- Complex wounds including burns, skin ulcers, and extensive wound debridement
- Acute exacerbations of neuromuscular disease processes
- Major gastrointestinal complications

As previously mentioned, patients with the above-listed conditions may require an emergent or planned airway procedure within the operating room, emergency department, or intensive care unit setting. An invasive or noninvasive intervention may be required depending on the 'algorithmic level' of the patient. Therefore, the clinician needs to be prepared and well skilled to overcome problems, as well as decisive when choosing interventions and avoiding futile interventions. A great number of fatal outcomes and irreversible brain injuries can be prevented by factors, such as detailed knowledge of the equipment available, proficiency in the use of this equipment, awareness of the time spent on the procedure, and finally the judgment to secure a timely surgical airway if necessary.

Emergency or urgent airway

Failure of awake-fiberoptic or GlideScope-assisted intubation may be due to tumor, secretions, infections (abscess, pneumonia, bronchitis), edema, trauma (maxillofacial, head, severe spinal injury), foreign body obstruction, trismus, rheumatoid arthritis (decreased range of motion), bleeding, or distorted anatomy (subglottic stenosis, mandibular hypoplasia, cervical abnormalities, large tongue or a cleft palate, obesity).

Trismus (<2 cm opening), in particular, predisposes to difficult airway. An opening of at least two large fingerbreadths between the upper and lower incisors is typically necessary for oral endotracheal intubation in an adult.

An emergency surgical airway is the final common resolution of any difficult airway algorithm when all previous attempts have been unsuccessful. The practitioner should be aware that persistent multiple attempts at intubation and poor technique are frequent common causes of delayed emergency surgical airway, leading to late poor outcomes.

Emergency surgical options include:

- Awake tracheotomy
- Cricothyroidotomy

The obese patient

Epidemiology

Worldwide, 35% of adults aged ≥20 are overweight, and 11% are classified as obese. It is estimated that at least 2.8 million people die each year as a result of overweight or obesity-related disease. More than one-third of the adult US population are considered obese, presenting a body mass index (BMI) of at least 30 (Ogden et al. 2006). Obesity has reached epidemic proportions globally and mortality rates increase with increasing degrees of measured BMI. In a large, nationwide US database review of 113,653 in-hospital adult tracheotomy patients, a mortality rate of 19.2% was observed in the obese cohort (Shah et al. 2012). Once associated with high-income countries, obesity is now also prevalent in low- and middle-income countries (WHO 2013).

Factors to consider in obese patients

Respiratory changes

The respiratory propensity for hypoxemia is due to a decrease in lung and chest wall compliance, resulting in reduced lung volumes. Functional residual capacity is reduced due to a decrease in expiratory reserve volume. OSA, obesity hypoventilation syndrome (OHS), and pulmonary hypertension can all be found within the obese population.

Comorbidities

Diabetes mellitus hypertension, heart failure, CVA.

Social factors

Lower levels of education, smoking, alcohol consumption, and limited access to health care.

Hospital-related factors

These include longer intensive care unit and hospital length of stay, lower rate of decannulation, increased risk of complications, higher accidental decannulation and false passage creation, and higher wound infection rate (Hogue et al. 2009, Cook et al. 2011).

Airway-related morbidity and mortality rate

In obese patients, increased delays are expected when securing the airway, combined with a tendency of the patient to develop hypoxemia faster and more frequently than nonobese patients. Therefore, the practitioner or anesthetist needs to successfully intubate and be able to ventilate these patients within a shorter period of time than nonobese patients, since oxygen desaturation places an additional strain on cardiac and pulmonary systems. Additional complications can be expected in this population, with presenting comorbidities related to obesity, including OSA, OHS, diabetes mellitus, pulmonary hypertension, and heart failure. Obesity and OSA are independent increased risk factors for 'cannot intubate/cannot ventilate' (CICV) patients. Although rare, this condition is fatal.

Different multi-institutional studies have demonstrated that tracheotomy and obesity itself are not directly related causes of mortality. However, the underlying comorbidities play a determinant role. These observations suggest that a careful analysis of risks and benefits will inform the decision to perform an invasive airway intervention in a critically ill patient with multiple comorbidities or a terminal illness. It is imperative to discuss the realistic goals of care objectively with the patient, their family, and the care team (Eibling & Roberson 2012, Shah et al. 2012).

Surgical airway in obese patients

Anatomical considerations

In obese patients, there is a reduced neck range (flexion/extension), which not only affects visualization by the anesthetist but also limits airway manipulation.

Since intubation is frequently more difficult in obese patients, it is important to be cognizant of when there is a need for an urgent airway. The surgeon must be aware that neck airway landmarks are not easily identifiable or present. These possible changes to the normal anatomy may require prompt adaptation to an effective modified approach to access the airway.

Such patients may also be at increased risk of aspiration due to upward displacement of the diaphragm by abdominal fat when in the supine position, displacing the parietal pleura superiorly. This poses a potential risk of pneumothorax, mainly in patients with COPD during surgical access. These risks can be decreased or prevented by the use of the 'sniffing the morning air' position. It was observed in a randomized, controlled study that preoxygenation in the 25° head-up position in severely obese patients achieved a 23% higher oxygen tension when compared to the supine position, thus allowing a significantly increased time for intubation and airway control (Dixon et al. 2005).

Cricothyrotomy in obese patients

This is a timely procedure of choice in any common final algorithm pathway for an emergent situation, when other initial maneuvers have failed to secure an airway.

- Stabilize the neck and palpate the skin to recognize landmarks in search of the depression from the cricothyroid membrane at the midline
- Clean the skin and infiltrate with 1% lidocaine with epinephrine 1:100,000 (0.01 mg/mL) at the site of the incision
- Probe deeply with the injection needle at the midline until aspirating intratracheal air, followed by spraying lidocaine into the tracheal lumen to reduce the cough reflex
- With the nondominant hand, immobilize the laryngeal cartilage with the thumb and third finger in a patient with recognizable anatomical landmarks on the anterior neck
- Make a 2 or 3 cm midline vertical skin and subcutaneous incision over the level of the cricothyroid membrane
- In an obese patient with a short neck and nonpalpable landmarks, make a 5 cm midline vertical incision and separate the subcutaneous fat tissue layer until finding strap muscles anteriorly and palpable landmarks (**Figure 14.2**)

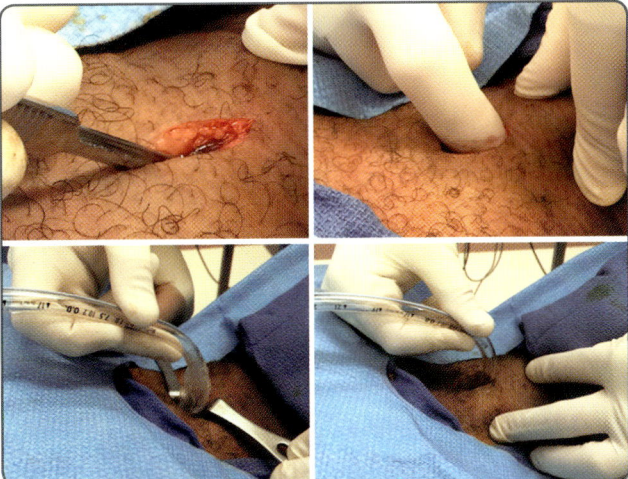

Figure 14.2 Cricothyrotomy with nonpalpable landmarks. Extended incision to separate subcutaneous fat tissue layer to find palpable landmarks.

- After identifying the midline over the cricothyroid membrane, incise horizontally about 1.5 cm at the lower aspect of the membrane where it is much less vascular
- Stabilize the lower thyroid cartilage with the cricoid hook, and introduce the Trousseau dilator through the incision and spread it vertically
- Insert an endotracheal tube or cuffed tracheostomy cannula #4, and gently inflate the cuff, then test the cuff for the lowest sealing pressure
- Wait for confirmation of the correct position of the tube, and verify effective airway re-establishment by expired end-tidal CO_2 monitoring or capnography

Once the patient has recovered and maintained in a clinically stable condition, a prompt reversal to a formal tracheotomy is recommended for two reasons. First, an endotracheal tube cannot be maintained safely in a stable position within the trachea for long. This increases the risk of accidental extubation, mainly in obese patients, resulting in higher chances for replacement into a false passage. Second, there is potential for the development of cartilage erosion due to trauma between the cricoid and first tracheal ring, progressing to subglottic stenosis.

Tracheotomy in obese patients

Chapter 5 outlines the standard tracheotomy technique.

A safer surgical approach is the same as that used for the obesity hypoventilation syndrome when prolonged or permanent use of tracheotomy is predicted (**Figure 14.3**).

These patients present a higher risk of accidental decannulation and the subsequent complication of false trajectory during replacement of the cannula. The use of a starplasty tracheotomy or other permanent tracheotomy technique combined with a generous anterior extended peristomal de-fatting has been suggested (**Figure 14.4**).

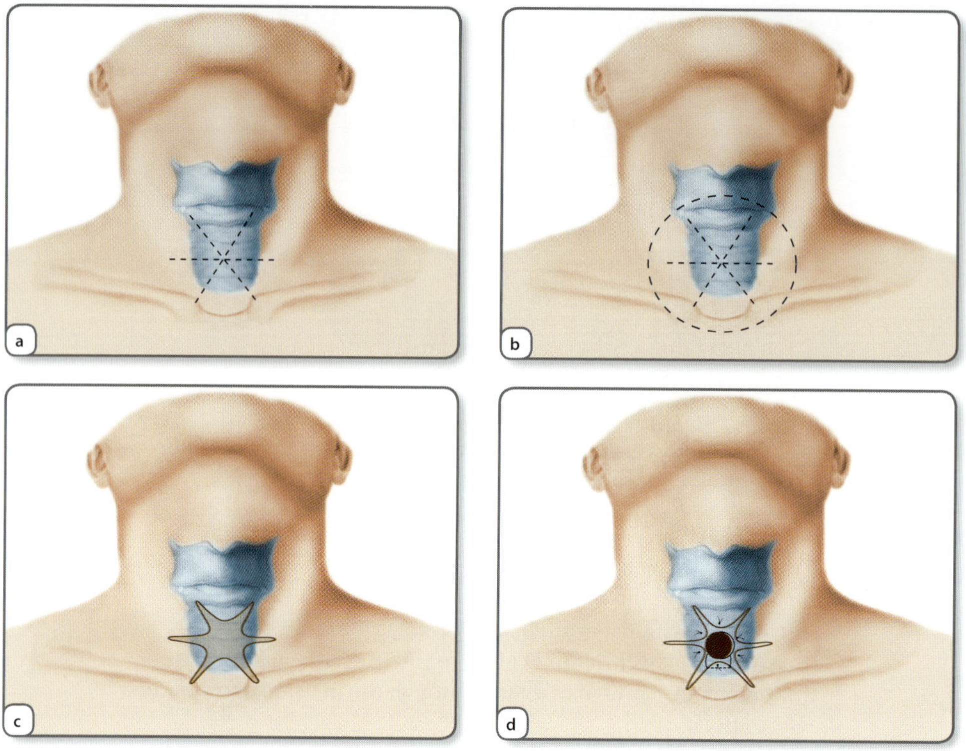

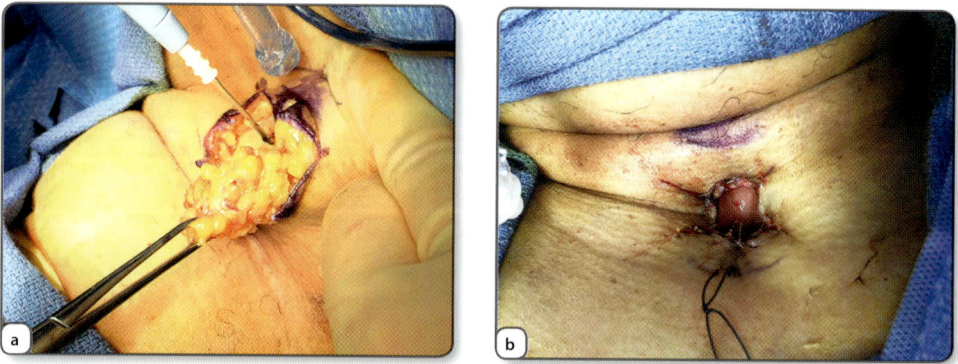

Figure 14.3 Permanent tracheotomy for severely obese patients. A sequential approach for the starplasty technique in combination with extended area of lipectomy. (a) Design of incision star shape with six flaps. (b) Circular demarcated area for lipectomy. (c) Extended lipectomy and exposure of strap muscles. (d) Peristomal flaps suture reconstruction and exposure of tracheal lumen.

Figure 14.4 (a) Peristomal extended lipectomy. Star-shaped incision with a large area of undermined subcutaneous fat tissue. (b) Final stoma aspect. This facilitates cannula manipulation and decreases the chances of false trajectory during replacement.

Post-tracheostomy physiology

The post-tracheostomy airway changes as a result of decreasing:
- Airway resistance, by passing air through a shorter circuit
- Cough reflex due to a decreased intrathoracic pressure
- Humidification, warming, and filtration of the air, causing thickening of secretions
- Movement of cilia, resulting in mucous plug formation and crusting
- Elevation of the larynx and incomplete closure of the vocal cords, causing aspiration
- Mobility of the larynx, contributing to dysphagia

Complications

The complications in obese patients are at least two-to-five times higher in the emergent airway situation when compared to elective tracheotomy (Gillespie & Eisele 1999). The surgical risk and complications increase exponentially when a critically ill patient with enlarged body habitus requires an urgent awake procedure. Complications can be classified as intraoperative (or immediate), early postoperative (until 1 week post-tracheotomy), and late postoperative.

Intraoperative complications
- Bleeding inferior thyroid artery, high-distorting innominate artery
- Laryngomalacia
- Unidentified subglottic stenosis from remote previous tracheotomy at a level below the sternal notch
- Pneumothorax: when there is higher exposure of the pleural wall on COPD/emphysema, decubitus in the severely obese or pregnant patient, progressing subcutaneous emphysema, previous lung surgery, and chest trauma
- Tracheomalacia: previous infection
- Unidentified enlarged thyroid gland

Early postoperative complications
- Mucous plugging
- Displacement of the cannula tip to the anterior or posterior wall of the trachea
- Accidental decannulation
- False trajectory of the cannula out of the trachea
- Surgical emphysema
- Aspiration

Late postoperative complications
- Mucous plugging
- Accidental decannulation
- False trajectory of the cannula out of the trachea
- Subglottic stenosis

Table 15.1 Types of percutaneous dilatational tracheostomy

Balloon-facilitated dilatational tracheostomy, Ciaglia Blue Dolphin	2005	Single-step dilation with balloon and loading dilator assembly, antegrade
T-Dagger, Amesh	2005	Single-step dilation with a curve, T-shaped dilator, elliptical in cross-section, ante grade
Dilating screw, Froval/Quintel	2002	Self-trapping screw, ante grade
Single-step dilator, Ciaglia Blue Rhino	1999	Single-step dilation with a curved dilator and loading dilator, ante grade
Translaryngeal tracheostomy, Fantoni	1997	Retrograde passage; specific cannula acts a dilator and tracheostomy tube
Dilating forceps, Griggs	1990	Dilation with specific forceps, ante grade
Sequential dilators, Ciaglia	1985	Multistep dilation with sequential dilators, ante grade

Table 15.2 Checklist for percutaneous dilation tracheostomy (PDT) procedure

Before the procedure:

Consent from the patient or family
Review coagulation studies (INR <1.5/ aPTT/Platelets > 50K/ No Plavix x 7 days)
Cease feed & aspirate NG/NJ tube (2 h before the procedure)
Preoxygenate (set ventilator FiO_2 to 100%) & set A/C mode, RR 12
TV 6 mL/kg IBW, PEEP 0 (if possible)
Increase threshold of the high-pressure alarm (100 cmH$_2$O)
Attach a capnograph to the ventilator circuit
Note: Bronchoscopy limited to confirm placement
(Guide wire and Tracheostomy tube)

Medications available at bedside (sedation, analgesia, and paralytics):
Infusion of propofol or midazolam
Fentanyl 200 µg before the procedure
Atracurium 50 mg or similar neuromuscular blocker
Xylocaine 1% with adrenaline 1:200,000 (local)
0.9% Normal saline 1 L for transient hypotension

aPTT, activated partial thromboplastin time; BMI, body mass index; INR, international normalized ratio

Percutaneous dilatational tracheostomy technique

Appropriate anatomical landmarks are identified, and the patient is premedicated with an intravenous narcotic and sedative (benzodiazepine or propofol). A paralytic agent may be given to prevent coughing unless otherwise contraindicated. The patient is preoxygenated with 100% oxygen, and the ventilator is placed on a set rate using a volume-cycled ventilator mode (**Table 15.2**). The patient is prepared and draped in a sterile procedure (neck hyperextension can be achieved by rolling two towels placed vertically under the shoulder blade to expose the neck/trachea, mainly after sedation and paralytics are given). Doppler ultrasound is currently used to identify patients (up to 20%) who may have large blood vessels crossing the landmark site in a vertical plane and who may therefore potentially develop significant bleeding during the dissection and insertion of the dilator.

Topical anesthetic with 1% lidocaine and epinephrine is given within the subcutaneous tissue and pretracheal fascia. A 1–1.5 cm incision is usually made 1 cm above the sternal notch. The horizontally incision is made at between the first and fourth tracheal cartilaginous rings. Blunt-dissection is used to gently spread the pretracheal planes and palpate the tracheal rings. A clamp is used next to apply pressure to the anterior tracheal wall, and to confirm the anticipated point of entry.

Bronchoscopy guidance helps to ensure proper airway withdrawal of the endotracheal tube to below the subglottic area. Bronchoscopy allows the PDT operator to identify the site of tracheotomy placement, gives direct visualization of the needle placement in the midline of the trachea, as well as allows identification of any damage to the posterior tracheal wall that may have occurred during the procedure (De Leyn et al 2007). The optimal position of the tracheostomy device should be between the first and second, or second and third tracheal rings. Percutaneous needle insertion should be between 10 and 2 o'clock in the visual field.

First, the introducer needle is passed through the incision and between the tracheal rings. The needle is attached to a saline-filled syringe so that air bubbles can be aspirated once inside the trachea. A guide wire is passed into the trachea via the introducer needle, and then the introducer needle is removed. A punch dilator is passed over the guide wire, creating the initial tract. A small catheter (white safety catheter) is then placed over the guide wire to prevent kinking of the guide wire (an indication of possible posterior wall injury). The large single dilator is then inserted into the trachea using gentle rotation. The tracheostomy tube is then preloaded onto a dilator/loader and passed over the guide wire into the newly established tract. Finally, the endotracheal tube is removed and the procedure ends after a bronchoscopic examination of the tracheostomy tube to confirm appropriate positioning within the trachea and the removal of any bloody secretions (Al-Ansari & Hijazi 2006).

Open surgical tracheostomy

Open surgical tracheostomy is usually performed in the operating room, where optimal conditions are provided for the higher-risk patient under general anesthesia. Each technique has advantages and pitfalls. However, certain variables will favor one over the other. Patient selection factors and the practitioner's expertise with the procedure will determine the most appropriate and safe procedure to follow (Freeman & Morris 2012).

Percutaneous dilatational tracheostomy versus open surgical tracheostomy

There are several advantages of PDT that explain its increased frequency of use in the intensive care unit when compared to open surgical tracheostomy. It is a less complex and more rapid procedure that can be performed at the patient's bedside, with faster scar healing. There are also advantages in terms of cost and safety, with a decreased incidence of wound infection when compared to standard tracheostomy. PDT avoids the risks and complications related to surgical intervention,

The TracMan trial, a large randomized study conducted in the United Kingdom, analyzed the influence of early tracheostomy (within 4 days of admission) on 30-day mortality, use of sedatives, and antibiotics in critically ill patients. The results showed no advantage in 30-day mortality or antibiotic administration in patients receiving early tracheostomy. However, patients were able to receive less sedative, even though this result did not change the duration of mechanical ventilation. In addition, the investigation showed no benefits with regard to the patient's extent of stay on the ventilator and/or in the intensive care unit (Young et al. 2013).

Despite controversial studies and results regarding the timing of tracheostomy, both options have specific indications, advantages, and complications. When the need for ventilator support is predicted to exceed a certain standard time (2 weeks), early tracheostomy is indicated. In this population, late tracheostomy results in an extended time spent in hospital and an increased chance of ventilator-associated events. Patients best suited to early tracheostomy are those presenting with neurologic and other conditions requiring special medical needs such as a spinal cord lesion (C4 and above), certain acute neuromuscular disorders resulting in respiratory failure, a poor Glasgow coma score by day 4, and patients who remain unconscious on mechanical ventilation for >3 days due to a supratentoria intracranial bleed.

In addition, upper airway obstruction, patients suffering from severe burns, or critical trauma cases involving the neck and upper airway are all indications for an early rather than late tracheostomy. The clinical decision to opt for early tracheostomy brings certain advantages, such as patient comfort, improved mouth hygiene, better pulmonary toilet, and an increased ability to communicate (e.g. using a Passy-Muir valve).

However, there is controversy regarding the advantages of early tracheostomy in terms of a reduced time on a mechanical ventilator, reduced time in the intensive care unit, and a shorter length of hospital stay. In addition, discussion is ongoing as to the correlation between early tracheostomy and positive outcomes on ventilator-associated events, use of antibiotics, sedation, and mortality in the intensive care unit. Despite all of these controversies, there is a tendency toward increased use of early tracheostomy procedures in the intensive care unit.

A providers' prediction of ventilator support duration is often inaccurate. Clinical reflection indicates that premature and unnecessary tracheostomy does occur, with unnecessary financial disadvantage and increased health risks. Questions remain regarding the consequences associated with the short- and long-term risks of having an artificial airway in the care of patients with respiratory failure.

Acute respiratory failure

Acute respiratory failure is a frequent diagnosis on admission to an intensive care unit and is a significant morbidity in the postoperative period in surgical patients. Mechanical ventilation as a support strategy is used to assist the patient with his or her work of breathing, to optimize ventilation in cases with CO_2 retention, and/or to help oxygenation deficits.

Acute respiratory failure occurs when there is an inability to effectively perform adequate ventilation, gas exchange, or when the burden of the patient's work of breathing challenges the respiratory pump to the point of fatigue (labored breathing). It is usually classified as hypercapnic or hypoxemic respiratory failure.

Respiratory failure subtypes

Hypercapnic respiratory failure

Hypercapnic respiratory failure occurs when there is CO_2 retention, which can lead to narcosis, an impairment of the level of consciousness. It is associated with an inappropriately low respiratory rate (e.g. with respiratory center depression as a result of opioid administration) or with ineffective ventilation [with a normal DO_2/Alveolar-arterial (A-a) gradient].

Hypoxemic respiratory failure

Hypoxemic respiratory failure is usually associated with an abnormally high A-a O_2 gradient (DO_2/A-a gradient) and can be secondary to ventilation/perfusion ($\dot{V}/\dot{Q}$) abnormalities [i.e. pneumonia, chronic obstructive pulmonary disease (COPD)], a shunt (i.e. acute respiratory distress syndrome) or less frequently due to a previously identified and known in the patient, a diffusion problem (i.e. interstitial parenchymal disease). The difference between $\dot{V}/\dot{Q}$ abnormalities and a shunt is a result of the ability of the former to respond to supplemental oxygen (FIO_2). Hypoxemic respiratory failure related to a shunt usually requires the use of PEEP ventilation to correct the abnormality (**Table 15.5**).

Clinical presentation and evaluation

Clinically, respiratory failure is recognized by evident distress or labored breathing (accessory respiratory muscles), changes of respiratory rate (tachypnea/or bradypnea), and/or cyanosis. The use of pulse oximetry (SpO_2) is valuable for the prompt, noninvasive bedside determination of hemoglobin oxygen saturation, which should be kept >90% if possible (using supplemental oxygen if needed). A chest

Table 15.5 A-a gradient (DO_2/A-a gradient)

A-a (O_2) gradient = $[(FIO_2\%/100) * (P_{atm} - 47\ mmHg) - (PaCO_2/0.8)] - PaO_2$

Where:
  FIO_2 room air = 21%
  Atmospheric pressure= 760 mmHg at sea level
  Water vapor pressure pH_2O (mmHg) = 47 mmHg at 37°C
  Respiratory quotient RQ (VCO_2/VO_2) = 0.8 (normal)
Normal range = 5–20 up to middle age (increases with age)
Expected A-a gradient = 2.5 + $[FIO_2\ (0.21) \times Age]$

X-ray, arterial blood gas analysis, electrocardiogram, and laboratory evaluation (complete blood count, chemistry, and cardiac enzymes) are simultaneously ordered upon admission to the intensive care unit of a patient with respiratory failure. The clinician should integrate all of this information to appropriately manage a patient with such a challenge. Noninvasive ventilation with combined pressure support and continuous positive airway pressure (CPAP) can assist mild clinical deteriorations until other pharmacological interventions take effect (i.e. furosemide diuresis in heart failure, aerosol nebulization in bronchospasm). More severe cases require the use of an endotracheal tube and mechanical ventilation.

Mechanical ventilation

When the decision is made to initiate mechanical ventilation, the airway needs to be secured, preferably with an orally inserted endotracheal tube placed by the most skilled available operator present using a laryngoscope, as it is imperative to prevent sustained oxygen desaturation in order to minimize end-organ damage. Appropriate positioning should be confirmed by immediate bilateral auscultation of Ambu-Bag-induced lung inflation, capnography, and later by a portable chest X-ray. Difficult airway intubation presents the medical care provider with situations that can be assisted by devices that give direct airway visualization (i.e. GlideScope, video endoscopy). Furthermore, the support of anesthesiology to provide deep sedation and/or transient paralysis is essential to secure the airway.

Mechanical ventilation requires several initial settings that the respiratory therapist should obtain from the physician for emergent operation of the equipment. These are (usually): Mode – assist-control (A/C); tidal volume – 6 mL/kg ideal body weight; respiratory rate – 12–15/minute; FiO_2 – 100%; and PEEP (5 initially). Consideration should be given to factors that may influence the initial and subsequent settings of these parameters.

Parameters that influence oxygenation

The FiO_2 should be decreased after the patient attains clinical stability to prevent long-term exposure to toxic levels of oxygen. The ideal scenario is to ventilate a patient with an FiO_2 of 40% if the conditions allow (SpO_2 ≥90%). The lowest possible levels of FiO_2 should be used for the shorter possible period of time. In order to use lower levels of FiO_2, it is customary to use increasing levels of PEEP. Pressures of 10 cmH_2O are usually well-tolerated in patients with adequate fluid status (volemia). Higher levels of PEEP are sometimes needed, but attention should be given to the impact of PEEP on the cardiac output (CO). The increased intrathoracic pressure may impair venous return and can decrease the CO. The use of PEEP is beneficial in the presence of bilateral disease with alveolar infiltrates (i.e. pulmonary edema). The clinical response to increasing levels of PEEP on asymmetric-unilateral disease is less predictable and can be deleterious by causing distension of the 'good' lung.

Parameters that influence minute ventilation

The $PaCO_2$ has a linear relationship with the minute ventilation (respiratory rate × tidal volume). The initial respiratory rate of 12–15/minute can be adjusted upward in patients with tachypnea due to increased work of breathing, systemic inflammatory response syndrome, or metabolic acidosis. The set respiratory rate could be as high as 70–80% of the patient's spontaneous respiratory rate. The increased respiratory rate will shorten the exhalation time, which in patients with airway flow limitation (i.e. COPD, or asthma) can induce an intrinsic-PEEP (auto-PEEP) that can negatively impact the patient's hemodynamics and decrease the CO. The tidal volume is set at 6 mL/kg of ideal body weight. The ARDSnet trial has shown that this setting is associated with better outcomes than the higher tidal volumes widely used previously by practitioners. The goal of ventilating with low tidal volumes is to secure a low mean alveolar pressure (plateau pressure), to reduce biotrauma and decrease the probability of ventilator-induced lung injury (ARDSnet 2000).

Other ventilator modes and factors

Pressure-controlled ventilation (PCV) has no proven outcome benefits over A/C. In clinical scenarios when lung compliance changes frequently, PCV will provide variable tidal volumes, which are a concern for the clinician. Pressure support (PS) is used in combination with CPAP and is a safe, acceptable, and useful technique of ventilator management. It is not used initially, but is a transition mode after clinical stability has been obtained (tidal volumes are not predictable by the level of PS) and to engage in a weaning process in patients with spontaneous ventilation. Synchronized intermittent mandatory ventilation has fallen into disfavor as it has been associated with worse outcomes when compared to the previously discussed modes. In patients with refractory hypoxemia, and in chronically ventilated patients, other useful mode techniques are available: proportional assist ventilation, neutrally adjusted ventilator assist, volume control plus, bi-level, airway pressure release ventilation, inverse ratio ventilation, high-frequency oscillation, and extracorporeal membrane oxygenation.

Aerosol therapy in tracheotomy patients

Aerosolized drugs produce a rapid pharmacological effect at lower dosages, with decreased complications when compared to systemic drug delivery. Tracheostomized patients receiving mechanical ventilation often require aerosol therapy through a nebulizer or a metered dose inhaler.

Weaning off mechanical ventilation

After the patients overcome the initial condition requiring them to need mechanical ventilatory support, they can be evaluated for weaning from ventilation if they have a reasonable level of consciousness and cooperation to manage their secretions, and if they can manage the extra workload with the use of noninvasive ventilation (NIV) if required. The rapid shallow breathing index (RSBI) is the ratio determined by the frequency divided by tidal volume in liters (f/TV) and is a time honored parameter, and a RSBI of ≤105 indicates a relatively low respiratory rate for an adequate tidal volume and is used to guide readiness for extubation (Yang & Tobin 1991).

If extubation is contemplated, enteral feeding and sedation should be stopped, respiratory therapy will provide maximal care (prescribed aerosols, toilette-suctioning), and the patients should be informed of the weaning-liberation trial to decrease their anxiety and gain cooperation. A minute ventilation of ≤10 L/min, the ability to maintain adequate oxygenation (SpO_2 ≥90%) without labored or distressed breathing or hemodynamic changes, and the ability to tolerate a low level of mechanical ventilation support (pressure support 5 cmH_2O and PEEP 5, or tube compensation) for 1–2 hours are all conditions that reassure the clinician of the patient's ability to be weaned from mechanical ventilator support. NIV can be used to assist patients in this transition and has allowed clinicians to shorten the duration of mechanical ventilation, reducing complications and ventilator-associated events (MacIntyre 2013, Penuelas et al. 2011).

General support of patients in the intensive care unit

Nutritional support (enteral), analgesia/sedation, prevention of hospital-acquired infection using care bundles (a group of evidence, e.g. head-of-bed elevation, oral chlorhexidine wash and body bath), and pharmacoprotection (ulcer, deep vein thrombosis prophylaxis, glycemic control) are key elements of care in modern intensive care units. More importantly, early mobilization, physical therapy, and sleep cycle protection are all interventions that will decrease intensive care unit-associated delirium and are increasingly being implemented as 'standards of care' in the intensive care units of hospitals with a recognized excellence of care (Jacobi et al. 2012).

Tracheostomy care

Appropriate care and management of tracheostomized individuals in the intensive care unit are imperative to promote the best clinical outcome. Implementation of tracheostomy care protocols is essential in order to minimize complications in patients with a tracheostomy. Recently, the American Academy of Otolaryngology–Head and Neck Surgery Foundation developed a clinical consensus statement. The study provides 77 statements covering all aspects of tracheostomy care, including ideal times for tube changing, necessary supplies, and care (Mitchell et al. 2013).

Physical therapy and mobilization in the intensive care unit

The benefits of early mobilization in the intensive care unit and its impact on functional outcomes need to be emphasized. The positive outcomes of early mobilization on muscle strength, length of stay in hospital, time on ventilation, and quality of life outweigh the otherwise minor risks. Mobilization should be initiated in the intensive care unit as soon as the patient is clinically stable, as reconditioning is an important part of tracheostomy care. Step-wise increments of patient turning, sitting upright in a chair, and walking are all important activities in pulmonary rehabilitation. Chest physiotherapy and postural drainage also play a role in improving tracheostomy care by facilitating secretion clearance (Adler & Malone 2012).

Conclusion

The intensive care unit is an experience that affects the patient in many ways and in many dimensions. The intensivist should consider the multisystem character of the conditions that bring a patient to the intensive care unit and should take the role of coordinator/leader of care among the other specialist care providers (nurses, therapists, and other physicians), the family, and the hospital medical system (i.e. faith support, administrators). Respect for patients' beliefs, culture, and desires should be taken into consideration in every decision relating to their care. Finally, the impact on long-term outcomes and the functional activities of daily living should always be in the mind of the provider, as post-traumatic stress disorder, quality of life issues, and cognitive impact form the centerpiece of current intensive care unit interventions and outcomes.

References

ARDSnet. Ventilation with lower tidal volumes as compared with traditional tidal volumes for acute lung injury and the acute respiratory distress syndrome. The Acute Respiratory Distress Syndrome Network. N Engl J Med 2000; 342:1301–1308.

Adler J, Malone D. Early mobilization in the intensive care unit: a systematic review. Cardiopulm Phys Ther J 2012; 23:5–13.

Al-Ansari MA, Hijazi MH. Clinical review: percutaneous dilatational tracheostomy. Crit Care 2006; 10:202.

Cabrini l, Monti G, Landoni G, et al. Percutaneous tracheostomy, a systematic review. Acta Anaesthesiol Scand 2012; 56:270–281.

De Leyn P, Bedert L, Delcroix M, et al. Tracheotomy: clinical review and guidelines. Eur J Cardiothorac Surg 2007; 32:412–421.

Dennis BM, Eckert MJ, Gunter OL, et al. Safety of bedside percutaneous tracheostomy in the critically ill: evaluation of more than 3,000 procedures. J Am Coll Surg 2013; 216:858–865; discussion 865–867.

Diehl JL, El Atrous S, Touchard D, et al. Changes in the work of breathing induced by tracheotomy in ventilator-dependent patients. Am J Respir Crit Care Med 1999; 159:383–388.

Durbin CG Jr, Perkins MP, Moores LK. Should tracheostomy be performed as early as 72 hours in patients requiring prolonged mechanical ventilation? Respir Care 2010; 55:76–87.

Engels PT, Bagshaw SM, Meier M, Brindley PG. Tracheostomy: from insertion to decannulation. Can J Surg 2009; 52:427–433.

Epstein SK. Late complications of tracheostomy. Respir Care 2005; 50:542–549.

Freeman BD, Morris PE. Tracheostomy practice in adults with acute respiratory failure. Crit Care Med 2012; 40:2890–2896.

Jacobi J, Bircher N, Krinsley J, et al. Guidelines for the use of an insulin infusion for the management of hyperglycemia in critically ill patients. Crit Care Med 2012; 40:3251–3276.

MacIntyre NR. The ventilator discontinuation process: an expanding evidence base. Respir Care 2013; 58:1074–1086.

Mitchell RB, Hussey HM, Setzen G, et al. Clinical consensus statement: tracheostomy care. Otolaryngol Head Neck Surg 2013; 148:6–20.

Peñuelas O, Frutos-Vivar F, Fernández C, et al. Characteristics and outcomes of ventilated patients according to time to liberation from mechanical ventilation. Am J Respir Crit Care Med 2011; 184:430–437.

Rumbak MJ, Newton M, Truncale T, et al. A prospective, randomized, study comparing early percutaneous dilational tracheotomy to prolonged translaryngeal intubation (delayed tracheotomy) in critically ill medical patients. Crit Care Med 2004; 32:1689–1694.

Shan L, Hao P, Xu F, Chen YG. Benefits of early tracheotomy: a meta-analysis based on 6 observational studies. Respir Care 2013; 58:1856–1862.

Simon M, Metschke M, Braune SA, et al. Death after percutaneous dilatational tracheostomy: a systematic review and analysis of risk factors. Crit Care 2013; 17:R258.

Trottier SJ, Hazard PB, Sakabu SA, et al. Posterior tracheal wall perforation during percutaneous dilational tracheostomy: an investigation into its mechanism and prevention. Chest 1999; 115:1383–1389.

Wang F, Wu Y, Bo L, et al. The timing of tracheotomy in critically ill patients undergoing mechanical ventilation: a systematic review and meta-analysis of randomized controlled trials. Chest 2011; 140:1456–1465.

Yang KL, Tobin MJ. A prospective study of indexes predicting the outcome of trials of weaning from mechanical ventilation. N Engl J Med 1991; 324:1445–1450.

Young D, Harrison DA, Cuthbertson BH. Effect of early vs late tracheostomy placement on survival in patients receiving mechanical ventilation: the TracMan randomized trial. JAMA 2013; 309:2121–2129.

Index

Note: Page numbers in **bold** or *italic* refer to tables or figures, respectively.

We view things from a certain position in time: in our language, thought, feelings and actions, we draw distinctions between what *has* happened, *is* happening, and *will* happen. Current approaches to this feature of our lives – those seen in disputes between tensed and tenseless theories, between realist and anti-realist treatments of past and future, and in accounts of historical knowledge – embody serious misunderstandings of the character of the issues; they misconstrue the relation between metaphysics and ethics, and the way to characterise the kind of sense which tensed language has. David Cockburn argues that the notion of 'reasons for emotion' must have a central place in any account of meaning, and that the *present* should have no priority in our understanding of tense. This allows for a more satisfactory articulation of the place of past, present and future in our thought, and of the form which criticism of our thought might take.